LYME DISEASE
The Untold Story

LYME DISEASE
The Untold Story

By
Dennis Allan Lakin

Phone: 1 / 888 / 888-7696

Printed in the United States

ISBN: 1-890622-15-X

Library of Congress Catalog Card No.: 97-076080

The views expressed in this book are the author's and are based on his experiences with this disease and his knowledge of science. This is not intended to replace competent medical advice.

TABLE OF CONTENTS

Foreword

Understanding the Author

"Where my Knowledge Comes From —Why the Doctors and Government Officials Don't Understand Like I do 1

My Experience with the Doctors and Their Receptionist........ 5

Six Main Problems with This Disease 41

I Saw the Light — My Mind was Filled with Information ... 60

The Main Things I've Learned about This Disease............... 63

The Symptoms of the So-Called Lyme Disease or DAL's Disease 66

How to Tell If You Have It When You Lay Down to Sleep or Wake Up in the Morning 87

The Squirrel and Rat Stories — Which Do You Fear? 99

Bear Hunting with Balls 106

Who the Millions of People Are Who Have This Disease and Where They Will Be Found..................... 110

Additional Information on Symptoms Taken from My First Book 117

The Kansas City Doctor Trouble Continues 123

Tell Them What They Want to Hear 131

The S.S.I. Adventure... 134

The Ultimate Nightmare — Held Hostage in America by a Foreigner 142

Photo Pages.. 162

Lyme Disease Symptoms in Toddlers................................. 167

FOREWORD

This book tells of a disease that is in America and other countries that very few people understand or want to accept that it even exists. But I know that uncountable millions of people have been exposed to it without knowing that they had or have it.

The doctors, along with our state government officials and CDC, though knowing little about this disease, have their stories of it.

I am no doctor, but I was an "A" student in science classes during high school. To receive "A" in any school subject means you know more about the subject or it is easy for you because you know it. So I'll describe myself as a scientist rather than a doctor.

When you read my book, you'll find I was a scientist who lived in the woods and laid on the ground without a house of shelter or public utilities. I did this three years through winter, spring, summer and fall, between the years of 1988 and 1992.

Therefore, when you hear the story of this disease from educated doctors or the CDC who wear suits and ties or white coats, their stories will differ from mine, because they were educated in a different way. When it comes to this disease, I didn't get my information of this disease from a book. "I wrote the book."

When I told my doctors that I was going to write a book about this disease (three different doctors in two different states), they all three looked at me and said, "You'd better do a lot of research before you start writing a book about a disease. I said, "No, Doc," I barely know how to read or spell. I'm not going to look up the answers. I know the story. I know what this disease does to the human body."

After I wrote my first book called "Lyme Disease — The Untold Story," I gave each one of them a copy (three doctors) and came back later to ask them what they thought of it. They all had the same answer, "It was interesting." That is all they could or would say about the book.

I don't think they liked the part of me telling the people how badly they treated me because I didn't have any insurance or money to pay them. That is all they were interested in — the money that I didn't have instead of the disease that I did have. They also didn't believe that I lived in the woods and laid on the ground without a house or public utilities in the 1990s.

I even tell the stories of the disbelieving doctors (greater detailed in this book.

What you are going to learn from my book is:

- The people who have this disease don't understand what is wrong with them.
- The doctors who treat their symptoms treat them with the wrong medicine, not believing that such a disease even exists and not wanting to admit to all the misdiagnosing done by the medical professionals.
- The word normal plays a very important part of this disease. When you don't understand the word normal, you don't understand what is wrong with your body, thinking arthritis, memory loss or nervousness is normal, no matter what your age.
- The person who has this disease has a very difficult time getting a doctor to believe that they have it, because they lose the capability of communicating. When you can't communicate or explain, getting a doctor to understand or believe you is so difficult.
- There are hundreds of thousands of misdiagnosed people who sit in nursing homes today in the 1990s who have been diagnosed with Alzheimers who really have this disease. Millions have died alone in nursing homes with this disease. The doctors won't tell you this because they are in cahoots with each other and fear malpractice suits. Other doctors just don't understand the symptoms.
- Millions suffer each day from arthritis who have been self-diagnosed, or misdiagnosed by the medical professionals who really have this disease.
- You will find that this disease plagues rural America and whole communities are infected, not affecting with as much fear. The inner cities like the dreaded AIDS virus.
- You will find out why our powerful government officials and our most educated medical professionals have no idea how widespread this disease really is.
- You will come to understand where these people who number in the millions who have this disease are located.

UNDERSTANDING THE AUTHOR

The information in this book was taken from the author's mind in a semi-conscious state.

It is written in his own words with the help of a higher power.

Dennis A. Lakin, the author of this book, has also written 10 small books on numerous subjects, such as: The Cookbook that Tells How to Get Rid of that Bigger Lower Belly; The Simple Dreams and Warm Love of a One-in-a-Million Man; P.M.S., A Man's Part, How to Help Your Mate; Arthritis, Alzheimers,Nervousness — The Untold Story of the #1 Cause and Cure; That Smoldering Cigarette; From Rats to Riches; The True Story of DAL; DAL's Advice on Winning the War on Drugs; and How to Be Both a Friend and Lover to a Woman. No matter who reads the books, they always describe them as original, or having never read a book like them before.

It may be due to the fact that Dennis isn't very good at spelling, reading or comprehending what he would read and has never made it very far through any book he has attempted to read.

Some educated people may say how can DAL write books if he can't read books. That is what makes his books different. As you will find when you read this one, this is a true story of his fight against a misunderstood disease, **a disease** that contaminated the inside of his body. He got it from exchanging bodily fluids with small, blood-sucking pests. Months before writing this book, Dennis couldn't:

- Use his brain to remember from one second to the next, what he did or where he went
- What year it was
- His age
- How to judge time, not being able to tell the difference between seconds, minutes or hours.
- He forgot the meaning of words and how to use words to

speak with, finish sentences or explain with.

- Didn't know what his house looked like or where it was located.

Not only having trouble with his brain, his body was also affected with pain from sore, tight, tense, tired muscles, and his joints were inflamed and locked up with arthritis. After going through this plus many more problems and symptoms, he says one day the **Lord God** showed him the light at the end of the tunnel when it comes to this disease, filling his mind with the information of it. He was told by the **Lord God** to share the information with the people of the world, to help them understand this disease and its symptoms.

He lost his brain's ability to figure out very simple things, though he could take some medicine and days later his brain would be clear-thinking once again. And his body's arthritic pain would totally disappear. He not only had a problem of this disease crippling his mind and body, he also had a problem getting doctors and pharmacists to give him medicine to treat his disease, because he didn't have any money, insurance or prescription. Dennis says he has visited the state of mind and body of arthritis, Alzheimers, nervousness and stuttering for weeks to years at a time, then returned back to the real world of normal people to tell of it, not once but over 10 different times.

This is his true story along with detailed symptoms of this misunderstood disease, caused by the tiny blood-sucking pests.

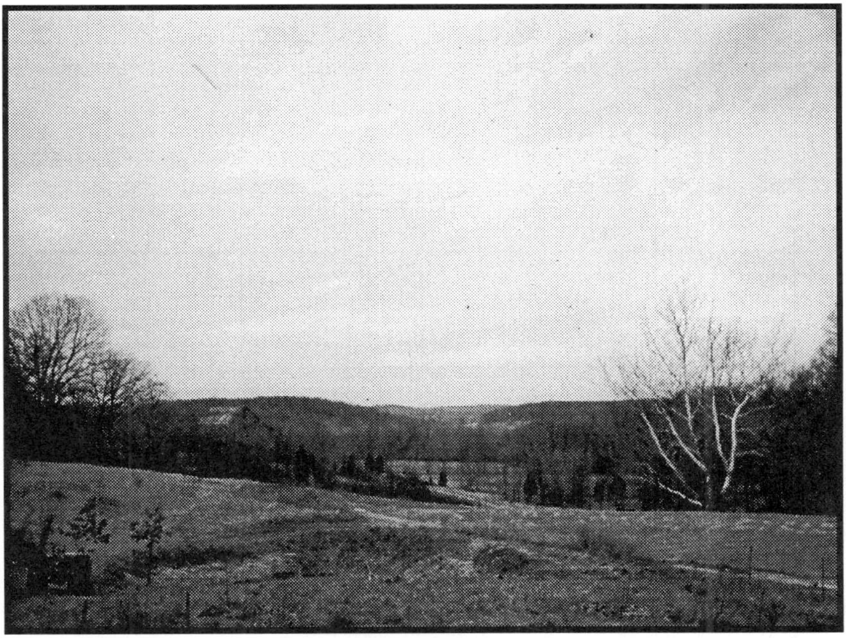

This was my front yard in the country where most of the story took place.

"WHERE MY KNOWLEDGE COMES FROM" Why the Doctors and Government Officials Don't Understand Like I Do

My dream has always been to live in the woods where there is nothing but trees, field and sky — a peaceful place away from the city life, some place where I could live in the woods and lay on the ground underneath the shade of a tree.

Well, I made it to that place, and always visited other peaceful places along the way years before. And I had no idea how dangerous blood-sucking pests were that lived in the woods and fields.

Pests such as: biting flies, fleas, mosquitoes and ticks. They all live there in uncountable numbers.

I didn't understand that they looked at me as food, and I looked at them like they were part of the outdoors. If I wanted to be there in the peacefulness of the outdoors, a couple of bites here and there by the blood-sucking pests didn't stop me from enjoying the beauty and peacefulness there.

Plus I'm a big tough guy. People are always describing me as Rambo or Clint Eastwood; why would a small insect scare me?

I used to lay in my field 20 miles from the nearest town in the middle of nowhere, in the night, surrounded by packs of yipping , howling coyotes and just stick my head under the sleeping bag and wait for them to leave.

I did it night after night and didn't think twice about it. If a pack of wild coyotes didn't scare me, what would make you think I was scared of small, sometimes invisible blood-sucking pests like chiggers or visible mosquitoes and ticks? They are so small. How could they hurt you? Or why would you fear them? Those coyotes are 60-80-lb. meat-eating wild dogs, and a biting fly, flea or mosquito has the weight of a small feather?

Which one of the animals would you fear? How about those doctors and government officials — which one do you think they are scared of? Probably both you and they would fear the pack of 80-lb. meat-eating wild dogs.

Well, I'm Rambo, and I fear the feather-weight, blood-sucking pest. **Think of it this way:** In order for those meat-eating wild dogs to eat you, they have to attack you, kill you, then eat you. As I look back on it, maybe I was too big for them, or they weren't hungry enough to mess with this Rambo. Or it could have been just one more time that the Lord God has His angel watching over me (probably a combination of all three).

Now for the tiny, nearly invisible blood-sucking pests. They look at a human being or animal and know all they have to do is penetrate their skin to get some food. They don't have to attack, kill, then eat. They attack and feast without killing.

You may think, **so what,** a biting fly bites me, or some chiggers, ticks, fleas, or mosquitoes. **They bite everyone, don't they?**

Yes, millions of blood-sucking pests bite millions of humans and animals every year. **So what … who cares …**

Well, I care, and I'm going to tell you something that may sound unbelievable but it's true. It's something that educated doctors and powerful government officials don't yet understand or won't yet accept, something that disbelievers in the Lord God may have a hard time understanding, too. But if you are a believer that Lord God does exist — let me start off by telling you that I truly believe in God and His son Jesus. Even though I'm described as Rambo, I'm a God-fearing man (which means to the layman who doesn't understand God that I'm afraid to do anything against God's teaching or will, because I fear the consequences).

So if I told you that the Lord God showed me the light and gave me the knowledge to warn the **world** about it, saying, "Don't worry about the doctors or government officials, they read their information out of a book, you write the books, then the believers will believe in you."

So take me very seriously when I say that for a human being to exchange bodily fluids with a blood-sucking pest is dangerous, and something to fear, **it's the truth!** Imagine the fluids from an insect's body being spit out into the human body's system.

You know of all the disgusting places and things flies hang around in, and the mosquitoes are born into stagnant water puddles; they lived on that water until they can fly. The bacteria from that water is inside them. It grows them. Fleas and lice could care less about what they bite as long as it's alive and has blood, and the bacteria from their family and their family's family is inside each and everyone, bacteria that came from birds, dogs, cats, rats, mice, etc. Their family's family sucked blood from all these creatures. You may wonder what is this Rambo-type of man so scared of that these insects carry.

Well, it's bacteria, the **spirochete**, that squirms and screws. And when this kind of bacteria breeds and grows inside the human body, it causes many cases of arthritis and Alzheimers, nervousness and stuttering.

As I said, the doctors aren't quite ready to accept this simple explanation of these diseases. And yes, many cases of arthritis and Alzheimers, nervousness and stuttering is a disease. **When taking the right medicine, they can be controlled. Arthritis pains vanish; memory returns to Alzheimers patients, and nervousness is gone from the nervous person, and the one who stutters may stutter no more.)**

You might think why don't they, doctors who went to school for years and have all that medical education, understand this. **It's because they went to the wrong school and read the wrong books** when it comes to this disease.

You see, I went to the school of hard knocks. I lived in the woods and laid on the ground through winter, spring, summer and fall months without a house of shelter or public utilities. I was bitten by over 4,000 ticks of all kinds and over 50,000 mosquitoes.

I forgot what year it was, how to spell my name correctly, what I did seconds, minutes, hours and days ago, whether my parents were dead or alive. My memory vanished. My body was so stiff and sore from arthritis I could barely walk or move; all I did was sit and stare. I was so nervous at that time I couldn't sit still, couldn't talk or explain to make any sense. All I did was stutter with nervousness, and couldn't use my brain to explain, to remember, comprehend or my body to move.

I didn't have money nor insurance, The doctors weren't interested in me at all; they were more concerned with how I'm going to pay my bills than they were in my health. Each time I'd say, "I have no money or insurance," their receptionists would say, "Well, we can't help you if you don't have money or insurance."

In short, my knowledge of this disease comes from experience and understanding of it. It's inside my body and won't go away. I live with it every day. I've visited the state of arthritis, Alzheimers and nervousness 10 times for months at a time, then returned back to the real world of normal people after taking medicine. I understand what the medicine can do for many of the people who suffer from arthritis, Alzheimers and nervousness. I guess you could also say if it wasn't for the doctor's receptionist who used to hang the phone up on me, I may not have entered so far into the late stage of arthritis, Alzheimers and nervousness, learning all I did about it.

I thank God for choosing this way for me to be heard and known.

MY EXPERIENCE
with the Doctors and Their Receptionist

I've told some of these stories about the doctors in my other books: **"Lyme Disease, the Untold Story"** and **"Arthritis, Alzheimers, Nervousness and Stuttering, The Untold Story of the #1 Cause and Cure."**

But I still have many more because trying to get a doctor to believe that this disease exists and that you have it is one of the problems with this disease. You know you have it, but the doctors disbelieve you and won't give the patients any medicine.

One of the reasons is the person with this bacteria in them has the symptoms of Alzheimers, memory loss, uncoordinated, incoherent, can't use their brain very well to concentrate, explain, visualize or comprehend. And this person is up against well-educated, **"clear-thinking doctors"** who disbelieve that this disease exists or that a tiny blood-sucking pest can actually cause these symptoms.

What happens is, after the first encounter with a clear-thinking doctor, the person with the symptoms of Alzheimers gives up trying to get medicine, because the doctors get them to believe nothing is wrong with them, and the person will either go away, thinking maybe "I'll just go to another doctor," and wait months and months to go back to the doctor again. Because of all the hassle, the **clear-thinking doctors** put them through, they think, *"I'm not going back to the doctor and have him tell me nothing is wrong. I'll just live with it. I know I'm not going to die yet,"* or they go from one doctor to another doctor before they find a doctor who will believe them.

Who do you think would come out ahead in an argument? The person with the symptoms of Alzheimers who can't remember what they did seconds, minutes or hours ago, having a blank cloud in their brain blocking their ability to concentrate or explain — or the clear-thinking, well-educated, disbelieving doctors?

It's no contest. The clear-thinking doctors will win the argument every time.

And that is what happens — hundreds of thousands of Alzheimers patients are being misdiagnosed and mistreated every year because of the disbelieving doctors who went to the wrong school and read the wrong book.

Here is what happened in my encounter with the doctors. (Let me remind you I knew exactly what was wrong with me except for the very first time). And I went in telling the doctors that I had it and what medicine I needed. Even with all this information, every one of them gave me trouble, because the clear-thinking doctor wins every time unless you are prepared and set in your mind that you are not leaving without a prescription to get some medicine.

But before I get into my stories, let me tell you two tricks I've found to work if the doctor is trying to send you away without medicine.

#1. Once you are in the room alone with the doctor and they're questioning and disbelieving all of what you are saying, you know they are not going to give you a prescription for some medicine. **You tell them straight out, "Doctor, I'm not leaving this room without a prescription to get some medicine,"** and sit and stare at them.

#2. Another more aggressive approach is to tell them if you don't give me some medicine, I'm going to catch you after work, walk up behind you and shoot you in the behind and blow your genitals off.

You usually don't have to do much talking after either one of these approaches, except to answer their question of what kind of medicine do you want and how much.

It starts off like this: I've lived in the woods and swamps all my life. I've been bitten by the ticks, mosquitoes, chiggers, biting flies and fleas all my life.

By the time I was 20, I encountered a few minor auto accidents and received whip-lash. Years afterwards, they never seemed to heal; my neck always hurt and was stiff. I had no strength, got head-rushes and had trouble with my memory.

So when I was 27 or so, I started going to a chiropractor school for treatment. Months before that was the first time I ever heard about Lyme Disease on T.V. They described all my symptoms, but I said to myself it's just my neck causing all those symptoms and my troubles. But since the intern wanted to take some blood for his grade in school, I asked him if he had heard about Lyme Disease. He said, "Yes ... it comes from ticks."

I said, "Well, I've been bitten over 1,500 times by the ticks and 50,000 times by mosquitoes."

He said he would just have my blood checked for that while he was out drawing blood. He said I could have it from being bit that many times.

Two weeks later the test came out **"Positive."** He told me I had definitely been exposed and had better go to a medical doctor and get some medicine.

I laughed at him and said, **"I'm not going to die, am I?"**

He said, "No, but you need medical treatment and had better get to a doctor quickly."

So I told all my buddies I had Lyme Disease. The doctor told me I did and that I had better see a medical doctor as quickly as possible. (I'm laughing about it, and they say I should not be laughing. I should go to the doctor **"Quick."**

I say, "Yeah." He says I'm not going to die, so I got time, plus I don't have money.

So three-four months passed by. I'm still suffering with arthritis pain, no energy and memory loss. I couldn't remember what I did from one day to the next. Then one day after a shower I was drying off and happened to look up in the mirror. As I strained to dry off, one side of my mouth was crooked. It looked paralyzed.

I told myself it's a "Bells Palsy," the late stage of Lyme Disease. I really do have Lyme Disease. I had better get to the doctor quickly.

So the next day I made an appointment. I told the doctor I had tested positive for it months ago and they told me to find a medical doctor, but I didn't.

So I go to the medical doctor. He gives me a three-week supply of medicine and told me to go to the hospital to have a blood test.

I tell him I don't have money for a test. I know I have it and I just need medicine. So I took the test and filled the prescription and started taking medicine. **(Three days later, I was walking down the sidewalk and I popped into reality.)**

All of a sudden I started to remember. I could remember what I did that day and the day before. I was now able to use my brain to remember. Before I couldn't (I never knew what it was like to be able to remember). I was amazed. The next thing I noticed: my neck didn't hurt any more. I had all kinds of energy, and all the arthritis pains in my body were gone.

I told myself I had Lyme Disease for years and didn't know or understand the symptoms. By the end of the three weeks of taking the medication I was a **brand new person,** with a brain I could use to think with and a body that moved again with no pains and was full of energy.

I was simply amazed now. I understood what it was like to be **normal,** like all the other normal people who could use their brains to think and remember, and had a body that didn't have any pains or run out of energy.

So with my amazing new body and brain, I excitedly called up the doctor to thank him.

The first thing I told him was how great I felt and how well the medicine worked.

He said, "Well, you didn't have Lyme Disease. Your test was negative. You have something else."

I said, "Something else? What else?"

He said, "Oh! It could have been anything."

I said, "**No,** I had it and I'm cured. I feel like a new person."

He said, "Your test was negative, and tests don't lie."

I said, "But the test before was positive, plus the side of my face was paralyzed."

He said, "No, you had something else. Your test was negative."

Then I finally realized this doctor didn't believe me, even though I told him my other test was positive and I felt a hundred times better.

All he kept on saying was, "The test was negative, and Lyme Disease isn't in this area. It's up in Connecticut."

That was my first experience with the disbelieving doctor, but I figured it didn't matter at all if he believed me or not as long as I'm cured, and that is what counts.

A couple of months after taking the medicine, my symptoms slowly returned but weren't so bad. I still had energy.

Then the next spring and summer came — more ticks and mosquito bites, and I felt the symptoms again coming back stronger every day.

No energy, memory loss, head rushes, body aching all over, sharp pains that came out of nowhere in my joints and tendons, hands and arms fell asleep easily.

I knew I had it again. So I called the same doctor back and told him, **"I have it again."**

He said, "You didn't have it the first time."

I said, "Yes, I did and I do again."

He said, "Your test was negative. They don't lie. You didn't have it. It isn't in these parts."

I lived in Granite City, Illinois, at that time but visited my land in southeast Missouri regularly. I told him I was bitten by over 200 ticks already this year and over 4,000 mosquitoes. He still didn't believe me and said I had better find another doctor.

So the clear-thinking doctor won the argument against the

person with Alzheimers symptoms once again.

I gave up trying to find a doctor for months. In the meantime, I was getting bit by more and more ticks and mosquitoes. My land was deep in southeast Missouri where the ticks are everywhere. I'd find 20-30 crawling on me every day and chopped them up with my fingernails, then squeezed them between my thumbnails and left the blood and guts on my hands and fingers. I didn't wash my hands before I ate or slept and would pick my nose or rub my eyes without thinking twice about the germs and bacteria on my hands. Within a couple of months my arthritis pain was so bad in my hands and my fingers I had to stop and rub them constantly. I'd drop stuff out of my hands 10-15 times a day. It would just seem to fall out of them.

At 28, I knew something was wrong but lost all sense of reality, and time stood still. All I'd do was sit and stare at the trees and fields. I didn't know what month or year it was. Never could remember what I ate even seconds after eating, couldn't visualize anything. I had to struggle to walk. I'd get head rushes every time I got up.

When I came back to my house in the city, I noticed I couldn't turn a light switch on or off, even on the second and sometimes third or fourth try. When I'd try to do this, my hand would crash into the wall and collapse my fingers, or my arm would get wrapped around the door jam as I passed, and I couldn't find or feel the switch.

I'd say to myself, *"I used to be able to do that. Three-year-old kids can turn off a light switch with ease. I had better get to the doctor before I can't do anything."*

So in this unreal state of body and mind, I tried to find a doctor who would believe and treat me. Let me remind you all this time I knew exactly what kind of medicine I needed to get better, but couldn't go to the drugstore and buy it without a prescription, a very simple form of antibiotic that cost $13 a month.

So then I started calling doctors, and at this time I couldn't remember words to speak with or finish sentences. The clear-thinking receptionist would be speaking so fast and wouldn't give me time to think. They always seemed to be questioning and disbelieving me. So after the third or fourth doctor I called, all seemed to keep asking the same questions.

By then, I knew the questions the receptionist would ask. It would be something like: "How do you know you have Lyme Disease?"

My answer was: "I live in the woods and I've been bitten by over 2,500 ticks."

Her next question: "What makes you think you have Lyme Disease?"

"Well, I can't remember anything. I have no energy and have a hard time trying to turn on and off a light switch."

"Where do you work?"

"I don't work, can't work and don't have any energy, can't remember anything to do to work."

"Do you have any insurance?"

"Me, no ..."

"How do you expect to pay the doctor bills?"

This is where they always had me, between a rock and a hard spot.

All I could say was, "Well, a..., and they would turn from nice to bitch and say either: "You better find another doctor," or, "We can't help you without money or insurance."

So on the fifth call to the doctors trying to find some help, I got smart because it's that end question that always got me **rejected.**

I started trying to use my brain to think of a better plan and come up with the answer. When they ask me where I'll get the money to pay the doctor's bill, I'll just lie to them and say I got a job and plenty of money. On the fifth call, she also asked all the same questions.

By that time I had all the questions memorized because this was my last chance. If it didn't work this time, I'd just give up and turn into a vegetable at 29 and let the government take care of me in an old folks home.

So she got to the question of: "How are you going to pay your bill?"

"I have a job." Then a sudden silence, and I thought what if she asked me what my job was.

But instead her next words were: "Can you make it Wednesday at 3 p.m.?"

I said, "**Yeah,**" hung up the phone and forgot what day and time she said. Two days later I called her back and said I forgot when my appointment was. She told me and I wrote it down and made it to the doctor's office. They called my name, and I went into the room, alone with her. (For those of you who read my other books, this is the Oriental doctor).

The first thing she did was start questioning me, saying: "So you think you have Lyme Disease?"

I said, "Ya, ya, yaa..."

"What makes you think you have Lyme Disease?"

"Well, I live in the woods and lay on the ground and have been bitten by over 2,500 ticks. I don't have any house or electricity. Ticks are always crawling on and biting me. I had it before. I know the symptoms. I got it again."

"What are the symptoms?"

"I don't have energy. I can't remember what I did or ate, or where I went. My neck hurts, my hands ache, my joints ache, my knee tendons hurt, I can't straighten my leg. I pop in and out of reality, everything looks unreal, like I'm not in the world."

She said, "You could have anything."

I said, "What do you mean anything?"

She says, "Lyme Disease isn't around here. It is in Connecticut — way up north. The ticks around here don't carry it. But before you get it, you have to be bitten by 10,000 ticks. It's one in 10,000 that carry the disease, according to what we read and study in the medical journals."

I said, "I've done be- be- be- been bitten by 2,500 ticks. That is close enough to 10,000, isn't it? How many ticks have you been bitten by?"

She said, "I've never ever been bitten."

I said, "I need some medicine. I can't get it without a prescription."

She said, "Well, we have to take a test first."

I said, "I don't have any money for the test."

She said, "I can't give you any medicine without a test."

Then all of a sudden I pop into reality, straighten up and start thinking and staring at her like: "If you don't give me any medicine, I'm gonna jump out of this chair and beat your head against the wall."

But then I think she got nervous and started saying something. All I remembered later were the words: "Well, I'll give you a prescription with enough medicine to last until the summer is over, because the ticks will still be biting you through the summer and fall."

She gave me a prescription for a six-month supply of medicine. I took it, shook her hand and said, "Thanks."

She said, "Take this to the front desk."

I stopped by there, and the receptionist said $30. Ten dollars, that's all I got, I don't get paid until Friday I told her, and it worked.

She let me out of the building with the prescription I'd been waiting to get for months. And I didn't have $12 to get it filled. I got the money somewhere.

Three days after taking the medicine I started coming back to the real world that everyone is in. Two weeks later all my aches and pains were gone. My memory was unclouded. I could think again.

I took the medicine for six months but ran out in the winter. My symptoms slowly returned again but didn't bother me until the next spring when ticks and mosquitoes started biting me again.

Then it started all over. My symptoms came on real quick — each day I had more and more. The symptoms got stronger and stronger. I knew I had it again. All the same symptoms returned.

So I went back to the Oriental doctor and told her I had it again. She started questioning me, with disbelief that I live in the woods without a house and don't have any money. She said I needed to take a test this time since I didn't take it last time. She said, "Lyme Disease isn't around here, and it's only in a certain kind of tick."

I said, "No, Doctor, all the ticks have it, because I was only bitten 30 times this time. I'm coming back early so that I don't go into the late stage again and cannot think or move."

She said, "I'll give you some more medicine, but go down and take the test."

Then I got a three-month supply of 250 mg. of a certain kind of antibiotic. I went down and took the test, and I knew it would come back **Positive,** because I had all the symptoms again.

Two weeks later she said the result was negative, I didn't have it. By then I took the medicine and was feeling great. All my symptoms had leveled back off after three months of taking the medicine. Many more ticks and mosquito bites. Two weeks later I ran out of medicine, and all the symptoms were back.

I went back to the doctor and asked her for a prescription. But she said my test was negative and tests won't lie. I didn't have it.

I said I had it, they just can't find it in the test, plus I heard on T.V. that tests are poor in detecting it.

She said, "I can't give you any more medicine."

I told her, "I need medicine, and I'm not leaving without it. When I run out of it, I can't think or do anything. I need medicine."

She said, "I think I know what is wrong with you."

I was thinking she's ready to give it to me, she understands now.

But then she says, "I think it's all in your head."

I said, "No, Doctor, it's all over the inside of my body, not just in my head. It's in my brain, clouding up my brain, but it's also making my body nervous and in pain with no energy.

But the doctor insisted, "It's in your head."

I told her, "Okay, fine. It's in my head, just give me some medicine for my head, and I know it will work on my body, too, whether you understand it or not."

She said, "You need another doctor."

I said, "I don't need another doctor. I need some more stronger medicine."

She said again, "You need another doctor."

I look at her and think: **"You dummy. All you need to do is write me a prescription so I can get some more medicine."**

I told her, "Don't send me to another doctor. I'll have to try to convince them that I have it. I don't have time to play games with doctors. My mind is slipping away faster and faster every day."

Then she said, "You need to go to a psychiatrist."

I said, "Can they give me any medicine?"

She said, "No, but they can tell you what is wrong with you."

I said, "I know what's really wrong with me. I've been bitten by too many ticks and mosquitoes and have a disease. I can't get rid of it and need to take medicine for the rest of my life."

She said, "No, I think something else is wrong with you."

By now my nerves were on edge, and I was sitting in a closed room with the doctor, and **I was just about ready to jump up and grab her by the throat and force her to write me a prescription for some medicine.**

I stared at her, thinking, *"I'm not leaving the room without the prescription."* I pop out of reality, and she's over there flipping her lips. I can't remember one word of what she's saying.

Then all of a sudden I hear the words, **"I can't give you a prescription."**

I pop out of the chair and say, "What do you mean you can't? You are a doctor, aren't you?"

She backed up in her chair and said, "I don't know what is wrong with you."

I could see that I scared her, and she told me to go and see another doctor.

I said, "Will it cost me anything?

She said, "I'll check." Then she called the receptionist to call the Community Counseling Center to see if they can get me an appointment and see if it will cost me anything.

I said again, "Can that doctor you call write me a prescription for some medicine?"

She said, "No."

I instantly say, "If that doctor can't write me a prescription, that is the wrong doctor to go and see."

She said, "You can go see him."

By then I'd calmed down and started thinking that she was going to send me to a doctor who can't write me a prescription. And then she's not going to give me any medicine. I told myself, "Maybe I had better be nice to her."

So I told her if I go to the doctor and he says that I need some medicine, will you give it to me?

She said she'd have to read the doctor's report first and give me medicine if it's recommended. So I went to the psychiatrist.

He said, "What are you doing here?"

I told him that I was sent by some other doctor to see if something might be in my head. I needed to come and see you for two sessions.

In short, his findings were: I needed a medical doctor who could write a prescription for some medicine. I needed a prescription from the doctor because it was illegal to get this medicine without a prescription or break in a drugstore and steal it. So I went back to the doctor and told her what the psychiatrist told me.

I decided not to leave her room without any medicine this time. After about an hour of waiting in the waiting room, I asked the desk receptionist: "Can I have some medicine?"

Then she answered that I needed an appointment to see the doctor. It cost to see the doctor.

I told her I was here last week. She knows who I am and what I need. Where is she?

She answered, "She's back there, but you can't go back there without an appointment."

By this time my blood was boiling. I was popping in and out of reality and ready to kill. I turned around and said, "Okay, set me up an appointment."

She said, "I can't set you up an appointment unless you pay off your last bill."

I was a split second away from jumping over the counter and grabbing her by the throat, then slamming her head against the countertop, but I still had some of my mind left, and it told me not to do it that way.

Then I said, "All she did last time was say I needed another doctor and sent me home instead of giving me a prescription."

She said, "If you want to see the doctor, you have to pay your bill off."

I said, "Okay, I'll get the money."

Then she said when I came back I have to be able to pay for that visit, too. I needed $60 in all. She moved over by the counter and the appointment book. I thought, "Now she is close enough to grab, choke and slam her against the counter. But should I do it or not?"

Then she blurted out a date and time, and I said to write it down for me because my memory is **real** short.

So I managed to scarf up $60, and for 10 days I waited to go back. I lost more and more of my mind and energy, always knowing all I needed was some medicine to think straight and it was difficult to get. On appointment day I went back to see the doctor.

She said, "What do you want?"

I said, "A year's supply of medicine."

She wrote a prescription for a twelve-month supply and handed it to me.

I said to myself, *"Is that it? She's not going to torture me with a bunch of questions before giving it to me."*

Then she said, "Is that all you want?"

I said with surprise, "**Yeah ...**"

She said, "Go to the front desk."

I said, "Thanks a lot, Doc," and shook her hand and walked out with amazement, thinking it's never been that easy before. Something must be up. I walked to the front desk, and the receptionist said $60. I gave it to her. I was standing there waiting for her to torture me. And all she said was, **"That's all. You can go."**

I said, "You mean I can leave that quick?" I walked out the door, thinking this must not be real, I must dreaming. I'd never been able to get a prescription that easily in my life.

So I went to the pharmacist and handed him the prescription. A couple of minutes later, he handed me a bottle of medicine.

Within a half hour after walking into the doctor's office I was walking out of the drugstore with some medicine. I was suspicious all day, thinking that I was just dreaming.

Three days after taking the medicine, I was back in a real world with my own brain and body. In a month all my senses were back. My mind was clear and my body was full of energy.

I took the medicine through summer, fall, winter and spring. I felt great, no problem with anything. That next spring I was bitten by more ticks and mosquitoes, but still had medicine. The bites didn't seem to bother me.

Then my prescription ran out right at the beginning of summer. The ticks were still biting me at least five times a day because I didn't yet have a camper trailer and tent. Every tick seemed to scare me because I had no defense against them. Then within two weeks of running out of medicine my symptoms started returning. No energy, muscle ache and pains, tensions, nervousness, joints popped and cracked when I woke up in the morning, and my memory was disappearing quickly. I started getting body rushes and popping in and out of reality.

I told myself I have it again. What I didn't understand at that time was that I was so far into the late stage of the disease before that I would have to take medicine for the rest of my life to feel normal and be able to use my brain and body normally like everyone else can.

So I decided to set up an appointment with the doctor because soon I wouldn't be able to use my brain to think and my body to move. It would be much more difficult then to do simple things.

I went to the town and called the doctor. But the receptionist said the doctor was on vacation and she wasn't sure when she was returning. I told her to set me up an appointment and I'd call back in a couple of weeks. She said that the doctor told her not to make any appointments until she returned.

By this time of year the seed ticks were out, and they look like a small black speck of dust of a pin-head size. I was sleeping in my clothes, and every morning I'd find about 5-10 ticks stuck on and full of my blood.

I was also going back and forth to Granite City, Illinois, and fishing in a spot that very few people know about because you have to cross a couple of stagnant swamps and then find your way through a shaded jungle of overgrown trees and hundred-year-old vines. This place was a perfect breeding ground for mosquitoes, and there were thousands and thousands in the shaded woods. They attacked you in swarms of a thousand or more. You could walk as fast as you could, but they would still follow you in swarms. As soon as you would stop, they would come from the thick black swarm in the air to attack you.

I was bitten over 500 times each time I visited the place. When I'd come out, I'd be all numb, tingly and nervous inside my body for 5-10 days after visiting that place. Then the nervousness would eventually level off, until I'd go back and it would start all over again because of the massive mosquito bites. What I didn't understand at the time was that I had contracted **encephalitis.**

My brain stem and the lining of my brain were swelled up, causing my neck pain, my memory to vanish and all the nervousness I had inside, the shaking and tingly feeling.

I had a combination of Lyme Disease and Encephalitis. I thought I only had Lyme Disease and couldn't get the doctor to believe me that I had anything because I couldn't remember words to speak with or explain. They thought I was crazy or lying. I had a healthy-looking, dark-tanned, muscled body on the outside and a brain that was blank. I couldn't remember what I did, where I went or where I was going. Then time stood still with or without a watch. I didn't know what time it was, if it was morning or evening time. I traveled from Illinois to southeast Missouri, two hours' ride, and I couldn't remember anything. One minute it seemed like I was in Illinois and the next minute a hundred miles farther in Missouri. There was always one thing I didn't forget, and that was what a STOP sign means.

I'd find myself forgetting what green and yellow signal lights meant and all other road signs, but when it came to a **red** stop sign or **red** stop light, I had my mind trained: never forget that means STOP.

I'd be driving down the road, and it seemed like every car was speeding past me. Everything seemed so slow. I was driving like one of those 90 or 100-year-old men or women on the roadway that hold onto the steering wheel, looking straight ahead and scared to death to go over 30 or 40 mph.

My buddies would say, "Put your foot on the gas pedal. What are you doing, riding the brake? Everyone is passing us up, looking at you and honking because you're going so slow. You drive like some old lady on the road who cannot see."

Everything seemed to be flying past me, and it seemed like my truck had wings. I knew it could fly at 30-40 mph because I was traveling so fast. I was in an unreal world where time stood still. I was off balance and uncoordinated.

Anyway, back to the vacationing doctor. I called back two weeks later. My mind was all fuzzy. I couldn't talk to make any sense, couldn't remember one thing I did during the day.

I asked the receptionist, "Is the doctor back?"

She said, "Yes, but she isn't taking any patients."

I said, "Did you tell her I called?"

She said, "Yes, but she doesn't want to see anyone."

It didn't make any sense to me. I said, "I need some more medicine, all my symptoms are back."

She said, "You had better find a new doctor, okay? Bye," and hung up.

The receptionist left me hanging on the pay phone in the middle of what seemed like nowhere without a mind to think with. **So I started thinking and understood what those people with AIDS must be going through when they are trying to find a doctor who will help them. I felt like a person with AIDS and nowhere to turn.**

So I gave up trying to find a doctor and went back to the woods with the sky, trees, fields and ticks. I got bit by another 70-80 ticks, and I could care less. I couldn't find anyone to help me. I was depressed, so I started praying for God's help.

Then something told me to leave the land and go to the town and get some food, then go to my other cabin 20 miles away.

I went to town, got some food and a newspaper, then went back to my other cabin where there is electricity. I read the paper, and there it was: **"Lyme Disease" lecture** coming to Perryville, Missouri. It says two local expert doctors will be there. **Free admission ...**

Just what I need. It's a week away. I made it to the place where the seminar was, and there were nothing but old people ages 50-80 years old. I stuck out like a sore thumb. There was a projector and screen in the front. Then finally the doctor came, a tall, skinny guy in a suit and tie, with a Rolex watch.

I thought, *"That's the doctor. He's got so much energy that he has probably never been bitten by a tick in his life. What does he know about ticks?"* He is followed by a pretty, dark-haired, dark-eyed, tall, slim woman in a nice dress, with diamonds and gold all over her fingers.

I thought, *"Who is that rich bitch?"* Then there was a short, chubby, half-bald, slow-moving guy who looked like an ordinary, non-aggressive, non-material person. He introduced himself: "I'm Doctor A. This is my wife, Mrs. B, and my associate, Doctor D. We're the leading authorities on the subject of Lyme Disease. We are here to answer some questions and make you aware of this disease."

So I listened, watching slides, and I could tell by the doctor's movements he wasn't interested in a one-to-one relationship. All he wanted was their money. It was obvious by the clothes and jewelry he and his wife were wearing. She looked like all she did was spend her husband's money. But the other doctor looked cool. He looked and acted like he had been bitten by ticks. I told myself I could relate to him. He told about his office and the purpose to all his patients. Then suddenly I heard from him, "We are here to help you even if you don't have any money or insurance, if you think you have this disease. We take non-paying patients for research purposes. We even have free samples of medicine for those people who have it."

I thought, this is it. This is where the Lord God sent me, to the doctor I need. I wrote his name and number. I called his office, saying, "I went to Doctor A and Doctor D's lecture about Lyme Disease in Perryville, Missouri. The doctor said he takes people without money or insurance."

But the receptionist answered, "Well, they have. But they aren't taking any new patients right now."

I said, "I need help. I've been bitten over 3,000 times by the ticks. I know all about the symptoms."

She said, "He isn't taking any new patients at this time."

I said, "I can help them understand the symptoms. I'm special."

She said, "Let me have your name and number."

I said, "I don't have any phone. I live in the woods and lay on the ground."

She took my name and said to call back later. I called back in a couple of days. She repeated that the doctor was not taking any new patients.

I said to the receptionist, "Did you tell him that I know all about the symptoms of this disease?"

She said, "Yes, but he is not taking new patients."

I said, "What are they out lecturing for? Just telling people that they know all about this disease and promising to take care of them."

She said, "He is all booked up. Go and find another doctor." Then she hung up on me. (That was my second experience with this receptionist. Just call her Receptionist L.)

So I gave up trying to find another doctor again. It was too hard. They didn't understand. I was so depressed and went to the woods to stare at all the trees and fields. I got bit by more ticks again and started to understand about the frustration of people with AIDS, how they feel when they can't get any help from doctors because the doctors don't understand their disease or want a bunch of money to treat them, but they can't work to get any money.

So another month passed. By now I was in a comatose state of mind. All I did was sit and stare and have a loud ringing in my ears. My mind was completely clouded and blank. I had no idea of what year or month it was. I couldn't remember my own name or how to spell it.

All I did was stand for hours because I was too nervous and tense when I was sitting down. I was in a comatose state of mind with a numb, tingly feeling. And time stood still. I could never tell if it was morning or evening time. I didn't know if the sun was rising up to begin the day or if it was sunset to end the day.

On a scale of 1-10, my energy level could barely hit a 1.

My head, back, arms, legs, hands, fingers, feet, every inch of my body was in pain. My mind and body were totally separated. I could never remember what my body did seconds ago. My mind couldn't get my body to move (I'll explain this later). Mind and body separation.

It's just like the Alzheimers patients. Their mind and body are separated. I was as bad as any person in the old folks home diagnosed with Alzheimers, except that I was 29 and knew what I needed to come back to the real world. I even forgot how to use or put words together. My jaw was clamped shut with tension, and I could barely eat. After five or six bites of food, I had to stop, breathe and rest.

When I visited the city, **I would be standing around with tenseness. When I had to piss, I'd just piss on the floor or the walls of my condemned house, or go to the yard. And I thought it was funny. I forgot about the outside world. I couldn't figure out if they pissed on the floor and walls or not. Now I know it's not normal to do that.**

My mind was really slipping away. Maybe I had better get to the doctor before I forget what is wrong with me and never return to the real world.

I was already in the vegetable state of mind. I told myself I had better go tomorrow, but I was wondering what day is it tomorrow ... it could be Saturday or Sunday. I looked around and started wondering what time of the day it was. Was it just the beginning of the day? Maybe I'd go today.

So I went into the trailer and changed my clothes. I went to my bed and said, "Maybe I'll lie down first and see if it's getting lighter or darker. If it's lighter, I have plenty of time." When I woke up, it was dark. So I told myself it must have been evening or maybe I slept all day. I couldn't remember, but it didn't matter. I had to wait for daylight.

So I was lying there, trying to think, and thoughts were popping in and out of my head. Then a second later, I could not remember what I was thinking about. All I could feel was my brain trying to think. And I started wondering where is my body. It was so numb and tingly all over. I couldn't move my arms and legs. I was paralyzed.

It was totally black and dark. I started wondering where I was. (That always happened to me when I'd wake up at night.) I had no idea where I was, where I went to sleep, even with light in the room. **I had no idea and thought I was in hell. Sometimes I thought the flying saucers were carrying me away. Other times I thought everyone was dead and I was the only one left on earth.** They were all weird feelings to wake up to. (But I remind you, I was usually so out of energy and comatose in the night when I was sleeping that I'd sleep through the night without waking up.)

Then it's daylight and I know today is the day. I've got to try and go back to the doctor and get some medicine, or soon I'll enter into a state of all loss of reality and forget what kind of medicine I need to take to make me better.

I made it into the town and called the Oriental doctor back. I could barely talk. I told the receptionist that no other doctor would see me.

She said, "The doctor won't see you. Find another doctor." Then she hung up on me because I'm talking so slow.

I called the expert doctor back and said I have Lyme Disease and need some treatment.

The receptionist said, "We will make you an appointment. What's your name?"

I told her and she remembered my name.

She said, "Didn't you call her a couple of times before?"

I said, "Yes ... I still need some help."

"You don't have any money or insurance?"

I said, "**No** ... I'm poor. I live in the woods, lying on the ground and don't have electricity."

She said, "I'm sorry, we can't help you."

So I gave up again trying to find a doctor and went back to the woods for three-four days with depression because I had no place else to go. Ticks were always crawling on me; I couldn't get away from them. I was living in the woods and fields without a house of shelter, electricity for lights or fan and water to bathe with.

My brain got more scrambled, my nerves were on edge. Ticks were always crawling on me. I was scared of them more than ever. I was ready to explode with insanity, but kept on coming back to the peacefulness of the woods, my own trees and fields. (That was my dream.).

After four more days in the woods I went back to town. I didn't have any money, so I was scarfing food out of the dumpsters behind grocery stores. And it was time to get a new supply of food from the rich people's trash.

While I was in town, I called the doctor again. Then the expert doctor's receptionist answered. I told her that I wanted an appointment with the doctor because I have Lyme Disease.

She said, "Okay ... can you make it on Thursday at 9:45 a.m.?"

I said, "**YES.**"

"Do you have any insurance?"

I say, "**NO.**"

"What is your name?"

Then I told her who I was — and she said: "Didn't you call here before?"

I said, "Yes."

"Don't you have any job?"

I said, "**No,** I can't work, no energy, plus I forgot what to do if I had a job. But I know all about the disease. Please tell the research doctor I'll trade him some information for some medicine."

She said, "Oh! We can't do that," then hung up the phone on me.

Then again, I was at a pay phone in the middle of nowhere without a mind trying to get a doctor to help me. But they hung the phone up on me. **I feel like the AIDS patients — lost, hope-**

less, having a disease with no care that the doctors don't have enough education on how to treat.

So I decided to go back to the Oriental doctor's office and stand around. I told myself they might get tired of me, then give me some medicine I need.

Early I went there. The doctor wouldn't come out until 1 o'clock. At the time, the receptionist seemed nice. I said I'd just come back later.

When I came back at 12:45 p.m., the doctor's office was full of patients, but the receptionist told me straight out: "I don't think the doctor wants to see you. Sorry, but she doesn't know anything about **Lyme Disease."**

I said, "I know all about the disease. All I need is a prescription to get some medicine. I know the doctor knows me and what's wrong with me.

I was standing at the front desk, and old people were coming in and out. It seems I was the youngest patient there. The receptionist said again that the doctor didn't want to see me. Then she said I'd **better leave.**

The two receptionists were acting like I wasn't there. I was staring at the old people around, and they were staring at me, too.

I said, "Why are the old people getting some medicine? Why can't I?"

The receptionist said once again, "You need an appointment first."

I said, "Okay, give me an appointment."

She flipped through the pages of the appointment book, then said, "We are all booked up."

I looked at her (like you bitch) and said, "Tell the doctor I'll be back."

I walked out, got into the truck, drove to the woods, collected my thoughts and said to myself that I didn't care if they got made or not, I need help. I went straight back to the doctor's office, walked in and stood around the front desk.

Then I said, "I'm back," staring at the two receptionists as if I'm ready to hurt both of them, then go looking for the doctor. But they say nothing, and they seemed to be scared of me. I didn't intend to be turned away this time. They were just staring at each other, both silent, keeping their eyes on me also.

I was too tired of being pushed around by the uncaring doctors. I meant business this time. (I figured I could plead insanity if I got into trouble.)

So I kept on standing there, looking mean and mad. When the doctor came down the hallway, I told myself it's my chance to get a prescription.

I said, "Hi, Doc. Remember me?"

She answered, "Yes."

I said, "I need some medicine. My prescriptions ran out."

She said, "You need an appointment."

I said, "But the receptionist told me you are all booked up for months," pointing at the receptionist who looks very scared. "And I need it now. I'm all nervous, cannot remember anything and have more pains. And I ain't leaving without one this time."

The doctor looked at both of the receptionists. They were stiff as a board and had fear in their eyes. She whipped out the prescription pad and gave me a three-month supply of medicine.

I told the doctor, "I've been taking medicine for three years and ain't cured yet. I need more than that."

She said, "You better find another doctor."

I said, "I will try ..." then walked out, jumped in my truck and went to the drugstore.

America shouldn't be like that. After getting medicine, I took a double dosage on that day. Then I thanked **God** that I hadn't hurt somebody just to get my mind and body back together.

It took a lot longer to feel more normal that time. It took two weeks, compared to three days when I took medicine before, because I was so far into the comatose state of encephalitis.

Now that I had three months' supply of medicine, the first two weeks I took a double dose (first prescription gone). I started coming back to the real world, but I wasn't all together at all. My joints stopped aching, my muscles stopped hurting and I had lots of energy.

But something was still wrong with my brain. My memory didn't come back like it should. My nerves seemed much more nervous. I couldn't sit still.

After another two weeks of taking double doses of medicine, my memory returned and I was able to remember some of what I did. But the day before everything was always blank. My nerves got much better, became real calm and relaxed, no more tension. The medicine worked after three weeks of taking it.

When I woke up one morning, I was back to normal. I could remember what I did the day before and could visualize once again. I could also talk without repeating myself or stuttering. I could eat food without my jaws getting stiff or sore.

It was a beautiful clear blue morning. I was walking through my watermelon patch. Looking up in the sky, I saw a flash of light. Then all of a sudden somebody started talking to me. As quick as the flash of light was there, it was gone. And my mind was filled with all the information about this disease**, Lyme Disease.** (But it is not time yet to tell you this story. I'm not done yet telling you about my experience with the doctors and receptionists).

A week after this it was time to get my last prescription filled. I was thinking, *"I'm about out of medicine again, and the ticks are still biting me. I don't have any doctor who will give me any medicine."* The last batch of medicine I took didn't seem to work well, and I couldn't figure it out. It was the same stuff. I was even taking double and triple dosages.

All of a sudden, one day my symptoms started returning. My neck was hurting, my muscles ached, head rushes returned. Everything was back. I thought the last batch of medicine I took was defective. It wasn't working any more.

Then I took it back to the pharmacist. He asked if I was keeping it in the refrigerator.

I said, "I don't have one. I live in the woods without electricity."

He said, "Where are you keeping it?"

I said, "In the truck on the dashboard."

Then he said that was the wrong place to keep the medicine. He read the label which said: **Keep in a dark cool place.**

Then I realized I was out of medicine again without finding a doctor. Soon I'd lose my brain and body again. I started praying but no answers. I called up the expert doctor again, figuring it had been close to two months. Maybe she wouldn't remember me (but I have a different story this time).

I said, "I've been seeing a doctor, but the medicine quit working. I need some different stuff."

She said, "Do you have any insurance?"

I said, "No ..."

Then she asked me, "Can you pay for the doctor's visit?"

I say, "I guess..."

She asked my name, but when she heard it instantly the phone went dead. She hung up on me. And I thought, *"She's a red-neck bitch."*

I went to the woods, very depressed. Ticks were crawling all over me. There was no place to walk or stand without getting ticks on me. So I just lay down on the ground and cried.

The doctors didn't want to treat me because I didn't have any money or insurance. I was rapidly losing the ability to use my brain and body once more. And no one wanted to help me. I couldn't get more medicine without a prescription.

I didn't have energy to work. I started thinking some doctor would probably trade me a prescription for some information I knew. I figured if they wanted money they could get it from somebody else, because not everyone knows about this kind of disease like I do. I'd been there and returned five times now.

I knew all about the symptoms.

By calling the doctor's receptionist and saying, "I don't have money or insurance, but I know all about the symptoms of this disease, and I wonder if I could trade the doctor some information about it for a prescription for some medicine I need."

I called about four doctors' receptionists. And they all said the same thing, "Oh! We can't do that. You need insurance or money to see the doctor."

Then I thought that ordinary doctors weren't interested in my knowledge. I planned to try the expert doctor again. Maybe they would have a different receptionist there. No, just my luck, Receptionist L. again.

I told her, "I don't have any insurance or money, but I know all about this disease and what it does to the human body." Then I asked her if I could trade the expert doctor some information about this for a prescription.

She said the same thing, "Oh, no, we can't do that."

By the time I finished telling her, she knew it was me again. Instantly the phone went click. She hung up on me. I was rapidly losing my mind again.

A couple of days later I said to myself, *"I'll try one more time to call the researching expert doctor. Maybe he will answer the phone."* But when I called early, it was the Receptionist L again.

I said, "I have Lyme Disease." As soon as she realized it was me, the phone went dead.

I said, "Okay, that's it." My brain was scrambled. I was nervous and mad. My plan was to walk in and punch the receptionist in the nose. Then I would go looking for the doctor to get some medicine. And if I went to the nut house, they would give me some medicine.

I went to the area where the doctors' buildings were. I asked the security guard, "Where is this expert research Lyme Disease doctor? I have something for his receptionist."

I saw he had a small six-shot 38 strapped on his side.

The guard says, "It's down there, five sets of buildings on the side. Want me to show you?"

I said, "No, I'll find it."

I went to the building parking lot. It was full of cars. Maybe I'd go in first and check it out. So I went in, and there were five receptionists sitting inside an open booth, and the room was full of people — looked like over a hundred. Most of them were old people.

Then I stood up against the wall across from the receptionist and thought, *"Which one is she?"*

They started wondering who I was and asked me if I need some help.

I pretended I was lost and looking for the receptionist. One of them said, "She is on break." I couldn't move with those words I heard. I popped into reality and started thinking, *"Where am I? Who are all these people? What am I doing here?"*

I was looking outside. I had never been there before and didn't know where I was. It looked like I was in an office building in the middle of the city.

I told myself, *"I'm lost."* I walked outside and couldn't find my truck. There were cars everywhere. I was standing there thinking, *"Where did all these cars come from?"* It looked like a sea of cars, and I forgot what mine looked like.

Then I saw the security guard drive by. He stopped and said, "You found it?"

"Found what," I said.

He said, "The building."

I said, "What building?"

He said, "Are you okay?"

I said, "Well, the parking lot filled up, and I can't find my truck."

He said, "I saw it over there by the trees," pointing at the only row of trees around. "Want a ride over there?"

I said, "Okay," and got into his truck.

He said, "I live in the country myself. I think those ticks make me lose my memory sometimes."

I said, "Me, too..."

As soon as we pulled up to the truck, I popped back into reality again, and everything came back to me of what I was going to do. Then I thought, *"How did I wind up riding with that security guard?"*

On the way back I started thanking God for being with me.

After that I moved back to Kansas City, Missouri. I used to live there. Closer to the city, I thought I'd go to the doctor the black people on welfare go to. I had some black friends there and a condemned house I still owned. It was in a $10,000-neighborhood. I knew it wouldn't be like the peacefulness of the woods, but the front yard was large with three big 120-year-old trees in it.

One of my neighbors said, "You're back... Where have you been?"

I told her, "I've been living in the woods and moved back to find a doctor."

She asked, "What's wrong with you?"

I said, "I got too many tick and mosquito bites. Can't remember anything, and the doctor won't give me medicine. I don't have money, I can't work, I'm too sick. I figure I'll go down here to the local community health center where all these black people go to get free medical treatment."

So I cleaned up the trash, dust and chased the rats away in my house, then moved in. I hadn't been there in four years. All I brought with me was some clothes, tools, paper, half a truckload of watermelons and my 9mm Berreta. I didn't have any lock on the door yet. I'm the only white guy in the black neighborhood, unloading a half truckload of watermelons into a condemned house without a lock on the door. And there was a gang of 4-10-

year-olds spear chuckers standing on the sidewalk in front of my house licking their lips. I got the feeling that they're going to try breaking in and steal my watermelons. I told myself I'd better go and get a lock for the door.

As I backed out of the driveway, the gang looked at me like, "You dumb white boy, this is our neighborhood and we play in that condemned house. As soon as your truck is out of sight, we are going to get us some **watermelons."**

So I hurried down to the hardware store. Then 15 minutes later I came back and found there were three watermelons broken in the front yard. I believed that the little spear chuckers got inside my house and broke my watermelons.

I went inside and found out of 30 watermelons, there were three gone. I went outside, and on close inspection of the crime scene saw they were all broken by the neighbor's chain-link fence.

Then the answer popped in my brain that the four-foot chain-link fence is taller than any of those little spear chuckers were. The kids were only two to three feet tall. What happened was they couldn't lift those big watermelons over their head to get them across the fence. They dropped the watermelons trying to do so. I saw that the little spear chuckers next door had done it. They were going to give me trouble.

Then five minutes passed, and I heard a small knock at the door.

Opening the door, I saw a gang of 5-10-year-olds, two to three feet tall, black kids who were crawling and standing all over my front porch.

The first thing they said was, "Can we have some watermelons?"

I said, "How do you know I have some watermelons?"

They said, "We don't know."

I said, "Then who broke those watermelons in the front yard?"

They scratched their behinds and said, "We don't know."

I said, "I'm the new neighbor, and I don't want anybody in my yard. **Get out of here."**

They looked around and slowly walked off. Then three days later, there were three to four small black kids hanging on the chain-link fence on their side of the yard looking at me with those big, sad dark eyes, looking like "we're hungry."

I said, "You want a watermelon?"

They jumped up and down and started licking their lips. I went inside and got them one and handed it over the fence to the biggest kid. Then I said, "Stay out of my yard."

Three days after that I came home. I saw there was a line of 10 or more little black kids in the neighbor yards looking through the fence. I got out of my truck, and they started jumping up and down, hollering, "Can we have a watermelon, can we have a watermelon?"

I said, "Who are you?"

They said, "We live down the road."

I said, "You haven't been in my yard, have you?"

They said, "No..."

So I went in and got them a watermelon and handed it over the fence. All 10 of them bunched together and stuck up about 20 hands and arms, saying and shouting: "Give it to me, give it to me."

I brought it back over and held it. I said, "Wait a minute. This is for everybody." I gave it to the biggest kid of the group and told him to stay out of the yard. He took it off then running, as all of them followed him, saying, "I want peace... I want peace... (The story goes on and on, but you get the point).

In short, I was there for a week, cleaned the house, chased the rats away, secured the house, scarfed a new supply of food from the grocery stores' trash pile. Then I was ready to go find the doctors and get some medicine. I put some of my dirty clothes on with holes and went down to the place where the black people with no money go to get some medicine. I walked in, and all I noticed were big white eyes looking at me from everywhere. Everyone was black, and I was the only white guy there. They were all staring at me like: "What are you doing here, White Boy?"

I went to the receptionist and said, "I need some medical treatment. I have Lyme Disease."

She asked my name and said, "Fill out the paper."

After filling out the paper, I took it back to her.

She said, "You need to go to the accountant first. You owe a back bill from there before. You have to pay that first. It's $90 back bill."

I said, "I don't have any money except I got only $5" (that is all it's supposed to cost to see a doctor).

She said, "You have to take care of this back bill first. Then come back when you get some money."

I was confused where I'm going to get some money.

She says, "You own a property, don't you? A house?"

I said, "Yes... but I live in a condemned house without electricity and loaded with rats."

She looked at me doubtfully as if: "You're white and don't have a job. You look healthy."

(I have a disease in the inside but not on the outside of my body.)

After 10 minutes of torturing questions by her, finally she let me go to the adult medical clinic. The whole room was full of black people. I was standing out like a sore thumb.

I sat there for one and a half hours being stared at by all dark-skinned people with medical cards. Then finally it was my turn to see the doctor. I told him I had Lyme Disease.

He said, "It isn't around here, is it?"

I said, "No... I used to live in the woods and lie on the ground. I've been bitten by over 3,000 ticks and 60,000 mosquitoes, and I moved here in Kansas City. I don't have any doctor and I need medicine." (I told him what kind of medicine I needed.)

Then he said, "You need to go and look for an expert."

I said, "I've done been there. What I need is some medicine. I need a year's supply." (I gave him one of my books and said, "Read this and you will know all about Lyme Disease.")

He said, "All I can give you is enough for 14 days."

I said, "I've taken over 6,000 pills in the past five years and still haven't gotten rid of the disease. I have to take medicine for the rest of my life to feel **normal.** I have all the arthritis pain, my memory fades in and out."

He said, "You need to go to an expert and arthritis doctor."

I said, "Okay, take this book, Doctor, read it, give me 14 days' worth of medicine, I'll be back." (Then I took the prescription and left.)

Two days later I got a bill in the mail from the Center for $90 and $45. Two weeks later I ran out of medicine. I went back to the doctor's receptionist. I told her who I am and said that I need more medicine. I told her the doctors know me. She asked him, and he sent me out a supply of medicine for 10 days.

A few days after, I planned to go back to the Oriental doctor. She knows me, and get me a year's supply of medicine. By then, I kept trying to make friends with her, because I told her someday I was going to the Philippines to get me an Oriental girl. I'm going to bring her back and visit her. Trying to win her friendship (it's a long, long story), sometimes she likes me, then sometimes she doesn't **(it was according to whether I had money or not).**

In short, I drove 350 miles back to southeast Missouri with some money. I got a year supply of medicine from her. And I was okay for a year. By that time I'd done some work. I saved some money and stayed away from the ticks and mosquitoes, but I knew even staying away from them, the disease would recur when I ran out of medicine.

So a month before I ran out of medicine I was working at a lady's house painting her house. I had known her since before, and we were friends (a black lady who reminds me of Oprah

Winfrey).

I told her about my problem and how I have had trouble with the doctors.

She said she knows a doctor around the corner from her house where people go — to get disability or prescription of upper or downer.

I figured out that I had money now; all I needed was a doctor who would write me a prescription. The doctor mentioned by this black lady sounded like the one I'd like to know.

So I went over and gave his receptionist my book and told her to give it to the doctor and I'd be back when I need some medicine.

It was first come, first serve basis. So when I ran out of medicine, my symptoms started to recur. I decided to go there early before my mind got too bad. I was the first one who arrived early. I went directly to the receptionist.

I said, "I'm the guy with Lyme Disease and need some medicine."

She said, "Sit down."

Within a few minutes I was called and met the doctor. I introduced myself, "I'm the one who wrote the book, **"Lyme Disease."** Did you read it?

The doctor answered, "No."

I thought, *"Here we go again. This doctor is going to torture me because I wasn't prepared to think of any answer."* I figured he had read my book.

He said, "How do you know you have **Lyme Disease?**"

I said, "I lived in the woods and laid on the ground for three years without electricity and house. I was bitten over 60,000 times by the mosquitoes and 3,000 times by the ticks."

He said, "What makes you **think** you have Lyme Disease?"

I said, "I don't have energy."

Then I told him, "If you would read my book, you would know why I have it and where I got it." This doctor looks like he just woke up from a three-day drunk or he was addicted to

codeine. His face was all swelled and unshaved and he had a beer belly. And I couldn't tell if he was white or black. He laid back in his chair like he was still asleep. He was acting like a prick. All of his patients were black, and I was white.

If you want to know more about this doctor story, it's in my video called **"Lyme Disease, The Untold Story, How to Tell If You Have Been Exposed."** (In short, he thought I was a narc trying to bust him because I was white and didn't want drugs, only medicine.)

These stories are only half of my experience with the doctors and their receptionists (True Experience).

So maybe if you are a doctor, congressman, government official or Oprah Winfrey or Murray Povich, this will give you a little insight to know about this problem. It's not just me.

Every time I've heard a story about Lyme Disease, it always starts off like: "The doctors wouldn't believe me that I had it," or, "I had to go from one doctor to another doctor to another doctor before getting treated." If you don't believe me, you can ask **"anyone"** who had or has Lyme Disease, especially the one who was in the "late stage" of this disease. Ask them if it's easily cured or if they have to take medicine for the rest of their life just to feel normal. I already know the story and the answer. But you people need to find out more. There is something else that you don't know. And it is that there are millions and millions of people in the USA that suffer from this kind of disease and don't understand the symptoms.

I myself didn't understand the symptoms until I took some medicine. And neither will the disbeliever or the people in denial that they have it. And now I know about them, the doctors who have no idea what are the symptoms of **Lyme Disease.**

The government described the symptoms in 30 words. My book will describe the symptoms easily understood compared to the government book. It's because the government has no idea that there are whole towns and communities affected with this disease, adding up to millions and millions of people who have it.

What will happen if the doctors have misdiagnosed and mistreated millions and millions of patients, **and the doctors or the patients have no idea of their misdiagnosed case because they don't understand the symptoms.**

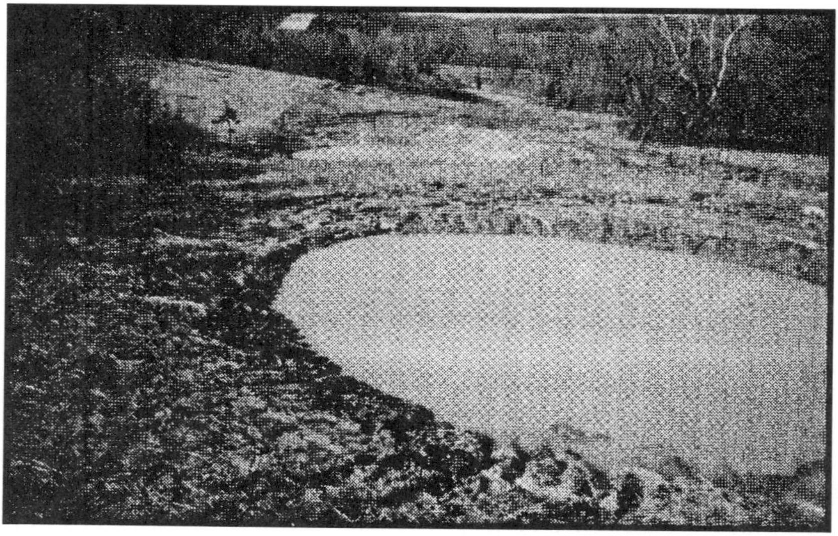

This is where my watermelon patch was located and where God filled my mind with the information on this disease.

SIX MAIN PROBLEMS WITH THIS DISEASE

1. **Government and doctors don't understand it or will not accept it.**
2. **Diagnostic test very, very poor.**
3. **The person who has it doesn't understand the symptoms.**
4. **Doctors very seldom report how many cases of the disease they did treat.**
5. **In order for the C.D.C. to file any cases of Lyme Disease, the bulls-eye ring has to have been present.**
6. **All the media people talk about is ... prevention.**

FIRST MAIN PROBLEM

Government and doctors don't understand it or will not accept that the so-called "Lyme Disease" exists. What they don't understand is that it has been here ever since the pioneers crossed America and way before that. One of the dumbest explanations they ever gave was that it migrated from Connecticut on birds, deer and mice.

If some of the government officials would have taken off their suits and ties and walked in the woods and fields, they would soon have realized that there are too many ticks that have always been here in America in the dense forest and fields, to make one ounce of sense out of those city slickers' theory. **This disease didn't just happen all of a sudden. It's always been here.** Some symptoms of it were just discovered.

These ticks move so **slow,** for them to get across one state it would take 100 years and generation after generation. So they didn't all of a sudden come down from Connecticut in a matter of a few short years; even to hop rides on animals would have taken 50-100 years, because animals are localized in their own area. **They don't leave their home and roam across the countryside.** And if it was on birds, birds would pull them off and eat them. (Birds are constantly cleaning themselves). So we will just say: **What a stupid theory the guys in the suits and ties have — who don't understand animals or survival.**

All ticks or at least 90% of them have the ability to give you this disease. **It doesn't matter what the government and the doctors say; they don't know the first thing about ticks or living in the woods without a house or electricity or needing medical help and not being able to get it.**

I know all about it; something else they don't understand is that all blood-sucking pests carry a form or relative of this deadly bacteria. Mosquitoes, biting flies, sand fleas, dog fleas, chiggers, lice and maybe leaches are a few more of the carriers of this disease. So it doesn't just come from ticks, but all kinds of blood-suckers.

Let me tell you a story about the fleas. I painted a young man's house. He was 28 at the time. This was three years after I understood about this disease. He had a good job, good insurance. When I first met him, he was always sitting because he had a hard time in walking. I asked him why.

He said that his joints were swollen up in his ankles and knees. It was painful to walk, joints swollen up and joint pain (the symptoms).

I asked him about other symptoms. He said he didn't have any except loss of energy. I asked if he had ever been bitten by the ticks.

He said, "No, but when I first moved into the house, it was infested with fleas. He got bit 10-20 times a night, mostly on the legs.

I looked at his ankle joints; they were swollen and his tendons were tight. I told him he had Lyme Disease.

He says, "What is that?"

To make the story short, I told him to take a test. He did, but it was **Negative.** The doctor was giving him anti-inflammatory medicine and shots of gold dust in his joints. **(Gold dust and insurance go together.)**

I said, "No, that is all wrong stuff. You need this form of medicine. Tell the doctor to give you some."

I left town for a couple of years, then dropped in one day when I was back in town.

He said, "I still have the same problem — joint pains." Two years later — now — other symptoms occurred. He could feel his heart beating all the time, got head rushes, etc. I told him to go and watch my video about the story of Lyme Disease. It was at the video rental store in town. I told him the fleas that bit him years ago caused him to have the so-called Lyme Disease.

He was still taking shots of gold dust. I came back and asked him if those were his symptoms.

He said, "Yes, those are my symptoms."

I asked him, "Did you get some medicine?"

He said the doctors wanted to keep giving him shots of gold dust; the insurance pays for it.

I said perhaps that doctor isn't interested in curing you ... all he wants is your money. Then I gave him a month supply of my medicine and told him I'd be back in a couple of months. Just take it regularly.

When I came back after two months, he and his wife were out digging flower beds in the front yard. I asked him how he was feeling.

He said, **"Great** ... no more pain. I can walk, run, dig, jump, and all the swelling is gone."

I said, "What did the doctor say about it?"

He said, "They don't believe that I'm cured and have no more pains."

I said, "Huh!!! Still going to him?"

He said, "I don't need to. He wants to keep injecting gold dust in a smaller amount.

I said, "Here is what you need to do. Go to another doctor and get a year prescription of the medicine. If and when you feel your symptoms returning, take it. Don't mess with that doctor. All he wants is your money. **(Gold dust ... what a joke.)** It's more like drain the insurance company.

So there is a proof that fleas carry it, too. There are millions and millions of people who have this disease in America alone. Millions and millions of them were misdiagnosed and mistreated years before the so-called Lyme Disease was ever heard of, from 10-100 or more years ago, when the ticks bit them when the cities were far and few in between nothing but fields, woods, sticks and mosquitoes. People have been being misdiagnosed for years and years with this disease. They sat in old folks homes from 10-20-30-40 years ago being diagnosed with Alzheimers, because the doctors had no idea what damage the blood-sucking pest could do to the human body. **(And they still don't understand.)**

Millions of people today in the 1990s sit alone in the nursing homes. They are diagnosed with Alzheimers, but don't really have Alzheimers. It's the late stage of too many tick and mosquito bites. When they were young, this bad, deadly, mind-and-body separating bacteria bred, grew and lived in them.

Let me share my knowledge with you of the late stage of too many tick and mosquito bites when left untreated: This bacteria will make at least two types of person: **The Blank Brain Person** and **The Scrambled Brain Person,** or they can be a combination of both.

In short, the Blank Brain Person:

- These types of people have a very low energy level, and time stands still for them.
- They just sit and stare.
- They can't remember anything.
- They look into the sky with their mouths open; they're in an unreal world, and time stands still.
- All they are seeing in their brain when they try to think is a cloud or blank picture.
- They will stare straight at you and see nothing but that blank.
- They will stare right through you without seeing anything. What is happening to cause that blank is the lining of their brain is

swollen along with their brain stem. And bacteria is squirming around in their brain tissue.

- There is a loud humming or ringing sound in their heads.
- Their tongue, throat or jaw muscle is locked tight.
- Their neck is tense.
- Nervousness occurs.
- Muscle twitching " it could be hands, fingers, a strand of arm muscle or leg muscle (a real thin strand hooked at both ends by tendons).
- It could be the eyes twitching, rapid eye movement (close and open).

These symptoms are caused by the late stage of too many ticks and mosquito bites. I'm the living proof. These were all my symptoms; that is why I know the answer.

If you know a person who has been diagnosed with Alzheimers, it could very, very, very well be the late stage of too many tick and mosquito bites left untreated. I visited this stage of mind and body more times than I care to remember. I only returned to the real world after visiting the unreal world by taking the right kind of medication.

So if you know someone with Alzheimers who has these very same symptoms who has left this world and is stuck in an unreal world, and the doctor says there's no way to bring them back to the real world ... **Hey** ... don't listen to them.

All you have to do is read my book called **"Arthritis, Alzheimers, Nervousness and Stuttering: The Untold Story of the #1 Cause and Cure.** It will tell you the medication that may possibly bring them back to this real world.

Now the Scramble Brain Person:

- May talk out of their head without making any sense at all.
- Jumping from one subject to another subject without finishing the subject or story.
- Ramble on, hit, slap, holler, yell.
- Can't be still or sit still, nerves on edge.

- Seems to be very nervous.
- Lots of movement here — not much pain or arthritis symptoms.
- Wide awake, full of energy with a scrambled brain.
- They are dangerous and aggressive.

Then there is a combination of both. These types of persons:
- One minute blank, then scrambled the next.
- These people are getting body rushes.
- Almost like a cold chill on the back of their neck, and it goes through their body creating energy.
- **Gained energy, then lost energy.**

Remember, the government and doctors don't understand this or won't accept it.

I'm not a doctor or government official, but I understand because I've been there. They won't understand and accept it.

Say it's the millions of misdiagnosed cases of arthritis that the doctors don't understand. This is much, much more common. **(You don't have to be a vegetable to have arthritis.)**

Arthritis is just one of the symptoms of this disease, and that is the only **noticeable symptom** you could have.

Millions and millions of people in the U.S. alone have **Arthritis** (40,000,000). I had it for years, and the doctor told me it was from a minor accident, and there wasn't a cure. I had the so-called arthritis for 12 years. I took this medicine, and three days later all my arthritis pain was gone. That is close enough to curable for me. It wasn't arthritis at all. It was too many tick and mosquito bites causing my arthritis. The doctors didn't understand it and neither did I. **But now I do.**

Millions have been misdiagnosed. 10-20-30-40-50 years ago, and still they are being misdiagnosed today in the 1990s. This means there are millions and millions of people suffering who have this disease and these symptoms of Alzheimers. We already have millions and millions of people exposed, and these are only two of the **symptoms.** The government says there are 17 symptoms in their books. But I know a lot more than 17, the ones that doctors, government and regular people don't understand. There is something else that the government doesn't understand, along with their friends, the C.D.C.

The C.D.C. started out saying that there are 10 cases here and 10 cases there. Then they went up to 100 cases here and 100 cases there. Then they went up to 500 cases here to 500 cases there, then to 1,000 cases here up to 1,000 cases there. Then 5,000 cases here, 5,000 cases there, then to 20,000 cases here and 20,000 cases there. Now they're up to 100,000 here and 100,000 there.

In a few short years what they don't understand or won't accept is: this disease plagues rural America, and there are millions and millions exposed. From years ago, these are just new cases they want to put numbers on. Whole communities and small towns are plagued with this disease, and neither the people, doctors or government understand it. Millions of people are exposed throughout America.

We have already established all these misdiagnosed cases of arthritis (millions) and misdiagnosed cases of Alzheimers (millions). Those are just two of the symptoms of this disease.

What about some of the others: Headache? This disease causes headaches that won't go away, a pain above the eyebrow on either side (migraine headache). How many suffer this?

Fatigue, loss of energy, no energy, can't get out of bed, can't move, sleep all day, no energy to do anything as: Chronic Fatigue Syndrome. Put the symptoms of Chronic Fatigue Syndrome together and what do you get? The same symptoms of Lyme Disease. And they don't know the cause and cure. It's because they got too much of the wrong education. They read it out of a book instead of studying it in the field of experience **(red-necks with college and book education).** Just like putting some country hick in the middle of New York City — what is the end result? He gets mugged or conned. The same with thousands of doctors with too much of the wrong education. What do you get ... millions of misdiagnosed cases of Lyme Disease or DAL's disease.

Irregular Heart Beat — what happens is you feel your heart beating when you are sitting, standing, lying still, or thickened blood beating through your veins, or you make a small move and your heart jumps a fast beat four or five times. **How many people go to the heart doctors and are misdiagnosed with whatever heart disease the doctor wants to name!**

Just a few more of the millions of misdiagnosed symptoms that the doctors don't understand because they went to the wrong school and read the wrong book. **Remember it could be only one noticeable symptom. This is a very important key to the disease.**

Mine started out with neck pain that didn't go away. That is the only one I noticed as a problem, thinking it was something else and it would never go away after 10 years of suffering.

Three days after taking the medicine, it was gone. I was amazed that that was really a symptom and it could be controlled to where it didn't bother me any more.

SECOND MAIN PROBLEM:

Diagnosed test very, very poor. (If the test is inaccurate, how can the true numbers exposed be accurate?)

In the early stage of this disease it doesn't show up in a test. You have to be in the late stage or have it for years before it **may** show up. Meaning **may** or **may not.** How accurate is that? Actually, for it to show up, the bacteria has to be in a countable number. In a small drop of blood before it gets to that countable number, it has to grow (meaning grow inside you).

I've taken four tests. Only the first one was **Positive.** The other three are **Negative.** But I still had it and still continue to have it.

No matter how much medicine I take to control the growth of this dangerous form of bacteria, once I stop taking medicine, it starts growing inside my blood again. It recurs again and won't go away. That is why in the early stage ... no matter what the test shows ... I'd take medicine anyway. Then if your symptoms are gone, you had it.

If the doctor says the test show you don't have it, demand that he give you medicine, not a two-week supply, but three-six months at least.

Here is another story *(a Research Biologist who was growing the bacteria for the state):*

I went to a Medical Center in southeast Missouri where they were growing the bacteria at a laboratory in test tubes and refrigerators. This was another one from the first encounter with the Oriental doctor. She gave me the address. *(This is a long story, but I will make it short.)*

I went to the laboratory, met the doctor and told him all about myself, that 2,500 ticks bit me. The first thing I noticed about this doctor was that he did a lot of staring into space and with his mouth open. All he did was listen to me talking and pick his nose. I knew he had it, right off. I told him about the symptoms, and he said he didn't have it; he had never been bitten.

But I could tell he had it by the way he stared into space with his mouth open and picked his nose at the same time. He was in the different world. He liked me because I knew all about the disease without reading it or going to school. He showed me a test tube and said there were 10 million live bacteria in it. Obviously he was playing with the bacteria, and now he is infected.

But this isn't the point. What I'm getting at is: he showed me some bacteria under the microscope. It looked like a stretched-out bedspring from a mattress with a screwing motion.

He said that is the stuff that causes the disease. On the way out, I told him I was writing a book about Lyme Disease and I would bring him a copy. I also told him that he had it; I could tell by the way he stared and listened without arguing.

I was just about done with the book (three weeks away). It would be printed and ready. (There is a story about him in it. He is the doctor who showed me the bacteria).

So I came back and gave him five copies of my book and told him to read it because he had the symptoms. I came back a year later with a video camera and asked him if I could talk to him for my video on Lyme Disease. And right off the bat, I could tell he read my book and found out he had it and got some medicine, because he was wide awake. He didn't stare into space, and he could talk and move **(not me telling the doctor that he had it is the point).** What I'm getting at is — he showed me the bacteria under the microscope again, and it was a totally different kind of bacteria. And he said that is the bacteria that causes the disease that comes from the tick's stomach. This stuff looked like squirming mosquito larvae. It was totally different. (You can see this live bacteria that causes this disease in my video mentioned).

The first time I saw it, it was six years after Lyme Disease came out in the news. They said that is the stuff. A year later he says something else is the stuff causing it. Meaning six or seven years after finding the disease they're not sure what the bacteria look like that cause it, even then.

So how can they make an accurate diagnosis or count the number of people exposed with the testing process ... when they're not sure what they are looking for? If they want to find this disease in numbers, it's not found in blood test. It's found in the symptoms. That is the very important key to this disease.

They can find it in the blood later, when they are sure of what they are looking for. For now, they need to treat the symptoms. If they go away, they had it. **That is what both the doctors and government need to understand with this new-found disease.**

THIRD MAIN PROBLEM:

The person who has this disease doesn't understand the symptoms of it, to know that they have a disease.

They think it's something else like:

- They slept wrong.
- They worked too hard.
- It's old age.

That was the same thing I thought, too. But old age at 20-30 years or even 50? A lot of what the person and the doctor blame on old age **isn't really old age. It's that their body is contaminated**

and broken down from a deadly form of bacteria inside their body from being bitten by the blood-sucking pest.

Just like the doctor who grew the bacteria, he didn't know he had it because he never was bitten by the ticks. All he did was play with the stuff and pick his nose. After reading my book, he found that this stuff could be going through his pores in his hand or up through his nose when he is picking his nose.

He opened my book one day after work, got suspicious of the symptoms, took some medicine and realized he had it. **What will happen with these symptoms is that they will distort the thinking of your mind into believing that nothing is wrong with you. By clouding up the thinking process, you just think it's just old age causing the problem, because the symptoms and pain are inside their body and they don't understand how anything could get inside there, causing the so-called symptoms of a disease.**

Note: This is a very misunderstood disease by the doctor and the person who has it.

Only I understand because of my entering the state of Arthritis-Alzheimers-Nervousness and Stuttering eight to ten times, then returning to the real world months later to tell of it. While I was there, I gathered information because I know all I needed was a certain kind of medicine to return to the real world. **It is now the people who don't understand what is wrong with them that I care about.**

Remember, I'm telling you that I saw the light, and the Lord God filled my mind with information about this disease. In that flashing second, I was also told with this information I was to warn and help people of the world with this problem, because millions have been misdiagnosed.

As of now, I have written two small books that tell of the symptoms of this disease and the danger of leaving it untreated. They are called "Lyme Disease — The Untold Story" and "Arthritis, Alzheimers, Nervousness and Stuttering — The Untold Story of the #1 Cause and Cure."

I've also made two videos on the subject called "Lyme Disease — The Untold Story — How to Tell If You Have Been Exposed" and "Lyme Disease — The Untold Story of Arthritis, Alzheimers, Nervousness and Stuttering," spending thousands of dollars to try to warn the people.

Now I'm sitting on the other side of the earth, in a Third World Country, on one of the islands in the Philippines, with my pretty new wife beside me. And the Lord God is guiding me to write this book. All the money I've spent doesn't matter to me. Money is only material wealth. My wealth is in faith and the Father who sent me to warn the people of the world of this danger.

Remember as I said in the beginning, if you are a non-believer in God, you may not believe in my knowledge. But I know my mission, and I trust my guide that I will always be guided in right direction.

Let me tell you about the most important thing I've found in the Third World Country that has America beat with hands down. It's not the fact that this place has a major pollution problem in the carboned-up jeepney, buses, trucks, motorcycles that have to go so slow because of all the people walking, standing and sitting everywhere along the roadway, or the fact that the inner city is polluted with plastic wrappers that once held food or water.

In other words, it is not that when these people get done eating something, they throw trash on the ground, or the fact that open sewer ditches drain along the roadways in front of everyone's house, and the smell of sewer drainage is everywhere. It is not the fact that the smell of deal animals rotting along the roadways is a good smell. What I like most about this place is: I can walk into any drugstore or pharmacy and tell them the kind of antibiotic I want or just write the name down on a piece of paper and hand it to the pharmacist. And they ask, "How many pieces do you want?" (Meaning, how much do you want?) **In other words, you don't need a prescription to get an antibiotic here in the Third World.)**

Now I'm talking directly to the congressmen and government officials of the U.S.A.

You can ask any woman who knows about a yeast infection

or has had one how important it is to start treating it at the first sign, not wait for weeks for a doctor's appointment to get a prescription.

One of the smartest things the government, F.D.A. (Food and Drug Administration) or whoever did it was to offer medicine for women who suffer from yeast infections over the counter. Now they don't have to wait and suffer if they think they have it. They go to the drugstore and buy the medicine over the counter or pick it off the shelf without a prescription. What a smart, caring idea!

I want to meet the person who had that law passed and shake their hand.)

That law will help millions of women who suffer from that infection here in the U.S.A. A lot of laws they pass are dumb, but that one was smart and directly to the sufferers.

What I'm getting at is that there needs to be a law passed here in the U.S.A. that is directed directly to the people who suffer from so-called Lyme Disease. When they feel those first symptoms coming on, they shouldn't have to wait and wait to go to the doctor before they can get some medicine, or have to deal with the torture of a disbelieving doctor, and slip further and further into the late stage of this disease.

The one who got the yeast law passed was probably a woman. And the one to get some kind of law for so-called Lyme Disease passed will not be a city slicker from the government or F.D.A., but a country boy in that office, one who understands what a tick is.

FOURTH MAIN PROBLEM:

Doctors very seldom report how many cases of the disease they did treat.

I learned this after being contacted by the Lyme Disease Association. I was featured in an article from a local newspaper called *The Pitch Weekly.*

The Lyme Disease Association contacted me, wanting me to come to their meeting they have once a month.

From the meeting I learned two things. One of them is: they

said that the doctors very seldom report any disease they treat to the C.D.C. because of all the paperwork that has to be done to do it. I know for a fact my disease was never reported to the C.D.C. because the doctors didn't believe that anything was wrong with me. Out of the 40 members of the association, they say not one of their disease cases was reported to the C.D.C. either.

So wake up ... how can the numbers they say there are be anywhere close to accurate? I know from the Giver of my gift (Lord God) along with the understanding of this disease that whatever number they say there is, it is many times more than that. I would bet any and everything I own on this statement. **I am so positive.**

FIFTH MAIN PROBLEM:

In order for the C.D.C. to file any cases of Lyme Disease, the bulls-eye ring has to have been present.

I also learned this at the meeting. I never had one except for a small 1/4-inch one after 500 more tick bites. There was only one person in the meeting who had one — one out of 40 infected people. How accurate is that? Those dumb red-necks in higher places just don't understand.

Let me tell you what I know about the bulls-eye ring from experience. I've always had a dark-tanned skin, just like many outdoor people and farmers who live with the sun). I never ever scratch my bites because I knew from watching the lighter, fair-skinned people of the country scratch theirs all the time, you get sores, marks and scars on your skin from doing so. So I never did. Dark-tanned skin is exposed to the sun — baked, hardened and less sensitive than the fair-skinned people. They scratch theirs, so the ring may appear more on lighter, fair-skinned people, sensitive-skinned people. **This is my only theory of the entire book. I will say this is a theory because I am not positive of this. But all else I say and have said is a fact. And I could care less who a person is or how much education he has that will disagree with me. There is no one here on earth who could ever convince me that I don't know what I'm talking about when it comes to this disease.**

Getting back to the C.D.C.'s filing the cases of this disease — those dumb red-necks just don't understand this disease at all. Clinical proof — Positive Blood Test — Bulls-Eye-Ring. They're worried about 3-5% of a hundred, and forget about the rest.

I'm worried about the 97-98% of the rest of the people who are infected and not counted in their numbers. They say you can't have this disease unless you have it their way. Diseases have no rules ... what kind of rules should a misunderstood disease have. Red-neck rules are just too strict for a disease that has the symptoms of 50 different other diseases.

SIXTH MAIN PROBLEM:

All the media people talk about is ... Prevention.

In short, prevention may be followed by 3-5% of the outdoor people **(mainly the scared city dwellers).** What about the 95% of the others? They know to do it — but do they? What a joke... people who live in the country would laugh at spraying themselves every time they stepped out the door. Could you imagine the inconvenience not to mention the cans of spray they would go through. These people live with the ticks and have for years. They already have the disease but don't understand the symptoms. And the outdoor man wear white clothing in the woods while looking for animals? Those animals aren't dumb. If only they could talk, they would say: "Look at this guy in the white clothing. He must be a city slicker, because he sure ain't no hunter dressed like that. I can see him from a mile away. He sure ain't going to sneak up on me. And the hunter knows this. Now I do admit the hunter will use spray.

But what about the others? What about the children? Children ... that rings a bell ... I have another story for you. Just as all my other stories, this is absolutely positively the **truth.**

I lived in a small community that used to be a summer resort, with cabins turned into permanent homes for many in southeast Missouri. After I came to understand this disease, I noticed that everyone down there had it (I mean everyone).

The owner's wife who now lives in California has been in an

old folks home diagnosed with Alzheimers for years **(what a coincidence).** One-half of this community are country red-necks, and the other half are cool. And ticks are everywhere as you enter this community on a gravel road.

The first resident just sits at a picnic table, stares into space with his mouth open. The second resident was bedridden. All he did was stare into space or at you and didn't know you, his family or wife, and would just lie there and shake with chills, and complained of pain. His wife (both were 20-year residents), nerves on edge. Talk, talk, talk, nervous, nervous, nervous, shake, shake, shake. (That's the only way to describe her.) Right there within a 1/4 mile of entry into the place, two Blank Brains and one Scrambled Brain person. It goes on and on — the younger ones have Arthritis and Nervousness. Everyone is infected but would never admit to it.

The kids by the time they reach kindergarten have been bitten by 500 or more ticks. By sixth grade they have been bitten 3-4 thousand times. Anyway, this story is about a couple. The man is skinny; the wife is chubby. They have two kids (2 and 6 years old). Through the summer months they are full of ticks. They sit around and pick ticks off each other night and day.

All the skinny man did was sit around with nervousness, picking his scabs and sores from the bites and shaking his leg and foot off the ground with nervousness. He doesn't talk a lot. But give him some beer, and you can't shut him up. He gets belligerent and dangerous. The true scrambled brain comes out in him.

The woman does nothing but stare into space with her mouth open and pick her nose, and is real slow with a blank brain in her response. (This story is actually about her and her denseness.)

His mom and dad, the only way to describe them is Arthritis pain and Nervousness. That is all they talk about their problem of these three words. **They are a combination of Blank and Scrambled Brains.**

The six-year-old girl had been bitten by ticks 800-1,000 times and dropped on her head twice from arm's height. She is nothing but hyperactive, can't sit still, can't stand still and won't shut up.

Her first year in kindergarten the teacher sent notes home all the time with her, saying she is uncontrollable, won't listen, sit still or shut up (need I say more), another Scrambled Brain.

Now the other one. This story is about the girl. The last time I saw her she was two years old. At the time she had been bitten by well over 300 ticks, could barely walk at two years old. All she did was stand up and wobble, then fall down on her head, face first or back first. This may seem funny, but to someone who likes kids it's probably not. This kid did nothing but stand up, wobble and fall down. And I don't mean fall down on her side or butt; it's her face first into the walls, doors, coffee table corners, toys or whatever she is near, she grabs for it, but if off by inches, she falls face first. I saw her fall out the door and down three iron steps 20 different times when I was there visiting them. I'd say she's going to fall out the door again. Her mom just sat there, staring at her with her mouth open. She fell out the door, bounced down the steps and hit the ground. On an average of three seconds later, the mom would close her mouth, get up, open the door and say, "Well, get up," to the crying kid.

Time after time after time this happened. She would also fall off the kitchen chair while crawling to the table, face first on the floor. The mom just stared at her and said, "Get up." This kid's face was full of bruises and scars. I know without a doubt I visited there and stayed overnight, maybe a total of 300-400 hours visiting at their house. The kid fell on her face well over 400 times. Imagine how many times she must have fallen in a year.

Now one more story about the falling kid. I was riding with them once and saw this three different times. The four of them were riding in the pick-up truck. I forgot where they went, but after getting back to their house and pulling into the driveway, the mom opened the truck door, and the two-year-old little girl fell out of the truck on her face in the gravel. I mean, just open the door and the kid falls out the door. From what I remember, the mother did this once, and the six-year-old other girl did it twice. The mother looks at the six-year-old girl and shuts her mouth and says, "You dummy, pick up your little sister." The little girl rolls over with rocks imbedded in her face, just screaming.

The slowness of the massive tick-bitten family — it may seem funny to some and I don't know what to others. All I know is — it is the truth and it was funny for me at the time when I was there. And I told myself if I write another book, I've got to tell of the family that used to open the truck door and let their baby fall out, face first.

I also have another story that seems funny that I always wanted to tell. I did this once when I wasn't in my right mind when I had Lyme Disease and didn't know the symptoms yet. But it's a long story. If I have room at the end, I'll tell it. It's about black bear hunting in California. With a can of mace, a mother, my Aries woman friend and her three kids. It was kind of dumb, and I wouldn't do it again without my 9mm hand gun.

Anyway, back to the Media people. Prevention ... that is all you hear. The main story is always cut short because they want to tell of prevention and of the C.D.C.'s low numbers exposed that are slowly rising. The way I see it, who cares about prevention — **surely not me. Have you ever read in any of my book about prevention. Definitely not.** I know all about this disease, and prevention is a waste of time in my book. I'd rather tell of my adventure with the rats, as you will come to find from reading the rats like me. Why would I worry about prevention? I already have the disease. It's inside my body, and it will not go away.

Prevention is used by the scared rich people who seldom go into the outdoors, so a $3 can of spray can last them a few years, or the outdoor man with a little money.

All the T.V. news and newspaper people are doing is wasting their time with prevention. In reality they may save 10-20 people from getting this disease. But the way **I see it** ... why worry about 10-20 people, when there are countless millions of people who already have the disease and don't understand the symptoms, or the countless millions who have been misdiagnosed by the doctors. They think the doctors can't be wrong because they went to school and read thousands of pages of medical books. What do the doctors know who went to the wrong school and read the wrong book, when it comes to understanding this disease.

That means they don't know anything compared to me. Remember I didn't read my information out of some book. **I wrote the book,** without looking up any answers. I possess a gift, not a bunch of hearsay. They say, "Follow these rules … don't say this … don't say that." You need all this book-educated research — **Baloney!**

Remember I left this world and visited the unreal world of mind and body that the doctors say you cannot return from. The information found in the unreal world isn't found in the real world. I was shown a way to enter the unreal world and return to the real world by a higher power, and was told to share my information with the believers of the world.

Remember the Lord God will take His children from this world (the earth) and leave all the rest (unbelievers) here on earth.

Just a short story: Years ago I met a brick layer who was married to a female evangelist. He was a drunk, and she was a preacher. While he was in the back room drinking whiskey, he told me many times he heard his wife telling of how God would some day come to take his children from the earth to another place. Why? Because the earth is actually **Hell.** Imagine not being able to go with God's children when it's time and being stuck on earth with all the evil destruction and bad people, at the end knowing you are stuck here forever and missed the chance to leave, knowing you are there for eternity and no way out. You are stuck with nuclear destruction and fires everywhere, no food, no water, evil everywhere. **You just remember when it happens, the guy who knows about so-called Lyme Disease also understands this (where Hell actually was). You will be saying why didn't I believe him.**

I SAW THE LIGHT, MY MIND WAS FILLED WITH INFORMATION

This story is for all the believers in the Lord God that he does exist

It goes like this: Starting out two weeks before I finally got some medicine, after stuttering and suffering for three or four months, slipping further and further into the late stage, this was the worst I had ever been.

- I lost all the sense of feeling.
- I was numb, tingly, shaky, tense, never could relax.
- All I did was stand and stare.
- It was hard to sit and eat.
- I'd sit down and pop back up.
- My muscles were twitching.
- I was dropping stuff out of my hands, it fell out. I couldn't hold on to it and couldn't pick up stuff. I'd reach for something and I couldn't reach it. If it was on the ground, I'd try three times before I could get it. I'd always say to myself, "Try again."
- When I touched something, I couldn't grasp it.
- My fingers didn't work, as if they weren't part of my body.
- All sensitivity was gone.
- I never knew what was happening with my body below my neck.
- I didn't know if it was morning or evening, when the sun was down or up in the sky.
- I couldn't judge what time it was.
- I couldn't tell if I had already gone through the day or was just starting to go through the day. Seconds seemed like hours. **In other words, I couldn't judge time. It just seemed to stand still.**
- I had no idea how to correctly judge a second from a minute or

a minute from an hour.

- Every muscle in my whole body was weak and in pain with every movement.
- I couldn't lift my arm above my head.
- My shoulder joints hurt so bad.
- The second I became conscious in the morning, my hips and legs would automatically tense up when I was awake.
- Uncontrollably my body was doing stuff that my brain hadn't told it to do.
- My brain had no idea what my body did, such as: I never knew where I went, where I was going, where I got back from, what I did.

I had a full plate of food, look at the plate when I was done, and I had no idea what had been on it, one second after eating. I'd watch T.V. and had no idea what was on. Couldn't think of the name or who the people were, such as: *Mash, Price is Right, Geraldo, Lucy Show,* any show you know by name. All looked like a comedy show or commercial. I couldn't tell a commercial from a T.V. series.

When I'd go to town or drive down the road, people were always staring at me. I think I walked like Frankenstein and drove like a grandma just staring ahead because of tenseness and blankness in my brain, and there was also ringing in my ears. Anyway, what I'm trying to get at is ... **I didn't know what was going on in the real world.** And I was in so much pain and out of energy I couldn't move and was full of nervousness and had no idea of it. The only words I could remember were: When asking a question ... "a - a - a - a - a, well - a - well a -" or when trying to talk, it's like "a - a - a - ..." or "I don't remember" or "I don't know." When I'd say, "a - a," I always ran into a cloud or blank in my brain and never could get around it. **That was my vocabulary at 29 years old because the doctors wouldn't give me medicine.**

Remember I know exactly what was wrong with me and what kind of medicine I needed to get better. In this state of mind and body, I planned to shot and kill the doctor's receptionist because I never could get past her on the phone to talk to the doctor to get some medicine. **Now out of the state of mind, as I sit back in the real world, I see that was a very dumb plan.** But when you lose the ability to use your brain on how to make a better plan, any plan is a good one. But as I see it now, "It wasn't **God's plan** for me to go through. He made a new plan for my life. I always ask Him to help me and guide me to the direction that He has planned for me.

Well, you know where I am now. He told me to leave the woods and guided me to the other side of the earth, gave me a beautiful wife. **And extended my vocabulary from "a - a - a," into writing all these pages of words to help the ordinary people of this world, along with someone who has the power and ability to understand and change what is not right.**

So the story goes: I described the state of mind and body I was in. I got some medicine and took it for three weeks. Later I came back to the **Real World.** It was about 9:30 in the morning, one summer day. I was walking across my half-acre watermelon patch. I went to the other side, turned around, looked up into the clear blue sky and saw a flash of light. I'm not sure if it was from the sky or just in my brain. But I heard someone speak to me, saying, **"You have the knowledge, use it in good faith."** And that was it. I was excited, thinking **God** is real. I tried to talk back, but there was nothing. No more words I heard. I was standing in the field next to my watermelon patch in the middle of nowhere with no one around for miles. I returned back home. I was in the real world on earth where all the other normal people are. From that day on, every time I'd enter the unreal state of mind and body (because of lack of medicine), I'd learn more and more about the **Disease.**

THE MAIN THINGS I'VE LEARNED ABOUT THIS DISEASE

Once you enter the late stage of this disease, it is difficult to return back to the same normal body and mind. It takes time — two to eight weeks of taking medicine. And most important, after you are in the late stage, you may have to take medicine for the rest of your life to feel good and normal. That is what the people who are in the early stage of the disease don't understand **— the ones in denial and the ones who have no idea that they have it.**

Taking medicine for the rest of your life is a regular job that costs money until you die. If you run out of medicine or quit taking it, all your symptoms return.

Remember, if you are one of the millions of people who have this disease, what you need to understand is that you could have only just one symptom and be misdiagnosed by the medical professional, saying you have:

- Arthritis
- Early Alzheimers
- Heart problem — feel your heart beating, pumping for no reason.
- Chronic Fatigue Syndrome
- Having stuttering problem
- Clogged or blank veins or arteries—if your hands, arms and feet fall asleep easily or feel your blood beating through your veins and arteries.
- Bursitis — shoulder joint pain when lifting arms.
- Tendonitis — tendon strained or pain.
- Calcified Elbows — that is what an old chiropractor diagnosed me with when I told him my hands and arms fell asleep easily when I'd place or position them above my stomach when I slept.

- Calcified Joints — stiff joints.
- Tennis Elbow
- Eye Allergy — that is how the eye doctor or ophthalmologist diagnosed me when I told him my eye muscle above always twitched and I saw an unreal picture.
- Migraine Headaches — this disease will cause headaches that won't go away, whether it be at the back of your skull, in the eyebrow or above the eyebrow.
- Flu or Fever.
- Nervousness — this usually comes in the late stage in the form of irritability. You get real irritable like:
  - — Want to snap at someone
  - — Can't sit still, can't stand still, go around in circles
  - — Can't finish your work
  - — Feels like you are doing a thousand things at one time
  - — Feels like your brain is ready to explode with irritability
  - — Shaking
  - — Jittery — inside your muscles feel like they are squeezing or shaking inside
  - — Stomach gets tight and tense
  - — Neck gets tight and tense

Doctors diagnose millions and millions of these cases every year, not knowing what causes them. Don't be misdiagnosed and come to find that you have it in the late stage years later, having to take medicine for the rest of your life ... just like me ... to feel normal.

Remember millions and millions have been misdiagnosed and continue to be misdiagnosed until these symptoms are accepted by the medical professionals, the ones who read the wrong book and went to the wrong school, the disbeliever who doesn't believe that a tiny, somewhat invisible, blood-sucking pest can actually cause the symptoms that millions and millions of people have.

I learned that the **doctors were wrong** who told me 15 years ago that I have arthritis and it can't be cured, telling me that I have to learn to live with it.

I learned that the **doctor was wrong** who told me my eye pain and twitching came from eye allergy.

I learned that the **chiropractor was wrong** who told me that I'd have to come and visit his office for months and months before he could start to make me better.

And the chiropractor who told me that I had calcified elbows **was wrong.**

I learned that the doctor who told me I didn't have energy because of lack of vitamins **was wrong.**

I learned that the doctor **was wrong** who told me at 26 years of age that I was getting old, and that was the cause of my aches, pains, loss of energy and memory.

I learned that there were uncountable millions of people who have this disease, that in no way did this disease migrate from Connecticut, wherever ticks are found. This disease is found, not just in one kind of tick, but in all kinds. And it is found not just in ticks, but all forms of blood-suckers carry a relative of this bacteria.

In short, all that I've told you I have learned about this disease, and it came from first-hand experience and from a Higher Power. I didn't need to look up my information as others did. My information was in the form of a learning experience.

I had this disease for 15 years without understanding the symptoms. Only after taking medicine did I understand that it was actually a disease causing all my problems and keeping me from being normal like other normal people.

THE SYMPTOMS OF THE SO-CALLED LYME DISEASE OR DAL'S DISEASE

This bacteria has attacked millions and millions of human beings, causing numerous symptoms. The medical professionals can't figure them out. They don't understand what causes these symptoms or why the human body has these symptoms.

But I know all about these symptoms. As a scientist, let's say a scientist who got A's and B's in Earth, Life and Biology Science and D's and F's in English, Math and History classes in high school.

A scientist who went to the other side of these symptoms, looked back at them, then returned to the real world to tell about it.

There is a scientific reason and answer why: Why is the sky blue? Why do the clouds with all that heavy water in them stay up in the air? What causes the pretty colors of the morning or evening sky before the sunrises and sunsets? These answers are all found in Earth Science Book.

But the answers to the symptoms that I'm going to describe are not found in medical books. That is one reason that the educated doctors don't know the answer and what causes these symptoms. They never found the answer in any book yet written here on earth.

These are the symptoms that the human body exhibits when its skin has been penetrated by blood-sucking pests, such as the ones I described.

These pests, while biting through your skin and sucking fluid such as blood from the human body, leave microscopic bacteria underneath the skin. When it penetrates the skin and under our sensitive skin is our system of body fluids that our skin protects, and when the pest penetrates the skin and starts feasting on the system, and when it gets full of our fluid taken from the body, it starts throwing back up into our system.

Example: Such as, if you suck on a straw or drink from a glass, when you swallow, some of the fluids from your mouth then go back into the glass or down back into the straw. It is mixed with whatever you are drinking.

When the blood-sucking pests are sucking your blood, when they are stopped or chased away by you or splattered all over your skin, the backwash that is in their mouth and stomachs are washed back or squashed back into your system. Imagine squashing a mosquito on you. It is stuck on you full of blood. The instant you slap and squash it before the blood squeezes out the side of its body, along with breaking its sucking tube off into your system, some of it is washed back into your system or the tick that stuck on you. It is small and flat. When it first bites and hooks to your skin and when it starts sucking your blood, it swells up getting fat and hard. When it is stretching its stomach to the limit, the backwash is put back into your system, or when you are squeezing a fat, blood-filled tick by the stomach, trying to pull it off from your skin.

Imagine you have a fat belly full of food and water. Some giant grabbed you by the belly and started squeezing. The first thing that will happen is you are going to throw up. That is how that deadly bacteria that causes the human body to suffer from these symptoms in the blood-sucking pest gets into your sensitive system underneath your skin, many forms and breeds of bacteria. (The Spirochete form of bacteria or Borrelia Burdorferi form is the most deadly).

- When it enters your body through the penetration of the skin; it's in your system.

- It continues to grow and multiply. These are the misunderstood and misdiagnosed symptoms that the contaminated human body exhibits. (If you want to see a form of this bacteria, it is shown in my video.)

What will happen to the contaminated person is:

- First your body will try to tell your brain that you have something wrong with it. Then later, your brain will try to tell your body something is wrong with it. **There is a separation of the brain and body. They don't work together.**

- Then the thinking process of your brain will be distorted into believing it's old age, because it's on the inside of your body, and you don't understand how it got there. **Remember, you may have only one or two of these symptoms for weeks, months or years before any other more serious ones occur.**

I had no idea that these were the symptoms of a disease. You can have only one of these symptoms and still have it without knowing or understanding it. I had only these symptoms for years. It was only after two years of massive mosquito bites and moving to the tick-infested southeast Missouri area that others occurred.

It starts out something like this:

- Sore, stiff, tired, weak muscles. When you are working on any job, doing anything, muscles puffing up, tense, weak with pain, cramp up. Your legs and back gets cramps while sleeping at night, tendon muscles are tight, side or back, tendon muscles are tense. **That is where the strands of muscles attach to the bones at the joint area.**

- **Twitching muscles.** Any area of your body may twitch uncontrollably for minutes to hours. Just one strand of muscle or a big chunk of muscle that flutters (mostly in legs, arms, stomach, shoulders, back). You can work for 5 to 10 minutes and your muscles that you use in working will be tight, tired and tense, where you used to be able to do the same things for hours without muscle pain, strain or tension at all. You may think, oh, it's old age, or they do that because I haven't used them in a while.

- **Neck pain.** I received whip-lash a few times that never seemed to heal. I thought this pain and tension would never go away. What happened was that deadly bacteria that entered my body was there waiting for a wounded, weak muscle to attack. It attacked that muscle squirming around in it, then inflamed it. Three days after taking medicine, the neck pain I had from those whiplashes for 10 years of suffering was gone.

  I'd wake up in the morning, my neck so stiff, tired, tense, weak and sore. Then about 10-11 a.m. the pain would start to subside, then come back later on. I'd have to lay down or go to bed early to ease the pain. It makes your neck real stiff, especially in turning side to side; it is really a problem. **It gets locked up with tension, and the flexibility is gone.** The pain and tension can be at the base of the skull, middle of neck or in shoulder area or in all three areas. You may feel fuzziness around the back of the head or back of your neck, get cold chills up your spine and neck. **This pain comes from your brainstem being swollen and the squirming bacteria inflaming the muscle, and sensitive nerves.**

- **Head rushes.** This goes along with the neck and swollen brainstem when you get up to move, whether your movement be fast or slow. When you get up, you feel a warmth going to your head, and it feels like you are going to faint. It's a dizzy, tingly feeling, blacking out feeling, like a sudden loss of energy throughout your body, and you have to stand still for a few seconds because of the blacking-out feeling.

  I had this problem for years and years, always thinking it was my neck out of place causing it. **But was I wrong!** After I took the medicine I never had this problem again, even with my cervical vertebrae out of place. But as soon as I run out of medicine or was bitten by another tick, it all comes back.

- **Body rush**. It's like a sudden loss of tingly energy or a swollen burst of tingly energy, a tingly muscle crawling, muscle twitching coming up or downburst. It can even be inside your chest or stomach. It doesn't stay in one area. It rushes up and down inside your body.

- **Headaches** (migraine headaches) that won't go away. It can be at the back of the skull, above the front of the ear, temple area, above the eyebrow area on either side. But it will usually be occurring on one side or spot, underneath the eyebrow area. A sharp, throbbing pain or dull ache usually goes along with the neckache or eye ache.

- **Uncoordinated or off-balance feeling.** My feet hurt on the bottom once I ran out of medicine. My feet became tender and felt like they had spurs on them — like knots. When I took some medicine it went away. Scared of heights — this goes along with the swollen brainstem and swollen brain lining. I used to fear heights because when I'd get up there, I'd be off balance. It felt like I was wobbling when I got close to the edge of a drop-off, a wobbling, swaying feeling. Then there's dropping stuff out of your hands and not being able to pick up something on the ground. The first and second try, when trying to do so, when closing your eyes you start to feel swaying, seasick movement, but when you open your eyes it's all right; the swaying stops.

- **You feel your heart beating** — or it feels like your heart is pumping thickened blood through your veins. You can be standing, sitting or lying, and you feel your heart beating with using no effort to do anything; it's just beating in your chest. Or you feel your heart jump or flutter. I had these symptoms for years, took some medicine and never felt my heart beat or flutter again until I ran out of medicine. **This is one of the first symptoms I noticed when the disease started to recur.** I can feel my heart beating when it's time to take some more medicine. (You see, you should never feel your heart beating.) After taking medicine I could run 500 feet and stop without feeling my heart beating, but without medicine I could run 50 feet, stop, and my heart was pounding through my chest. **That's a big difference and a very important symptom.**

This is a symptom that is very important. And if you think you have this disease, this is a way that you can tell yourself, because your heart is inside your body. Most noticeably it's when you lie down at night or to rest your heart is just pounding away inside your chest, a very simple sign and symptom. I felt my heart pounding for years and always jumped at the slightest little thing that scared me.

After taking medicine, I could run about the block, jump up and down for five minutes, and still couldn't feel my heart pounding. Before, all I had to do was stand up and my heart went Pa-boom — Pa-boom — Pa-boom. An amazingly big difference!

- **Nervousness.** This is also a very important symptom. How many people in the U.S.A. have been diagnosed by a doctor or just self-diagnosed with nervousness. Think of it this way: how did those nerves get damaged or short-circuited. How can you damage nerves inside your body? The only way to damage them would be to cut or crush them.

How This Disease Does It — It's with that Squirming Deadly Bad Bacteria

It squirms around inside your system, lays up against or hits up against the sensitive nervous system of our bodies and makes the nerves short circuited, making your nerves tense, jittery and shaky, on edge, irritable.

Have you ever seen an old person in an old folks home shaking with nervousness? How did their nerves with a system that has one of the strongest lining around it get damaged? It's not really damaged, but it's short circuited with this deadly form of bacteria that is laying up against their nerves.

What if you would ask one of the doctors that went to school for years why the old people shake?

Their answer would be something like: "It's **old age.** It's their nerves. It's their disease," or more likely they would just say, **"I don't know,"** or **"We are not sure." (which means they have no idea what is going on because they have never entered that state and returned to tell about it)**. They have never been close to being a vegetable in their life. But you know it from my writing how close I was to a nervous vegetable.

Eye twitching or eye pain deep and behind the eye. I went to an eye doctor. I wore glasses, and I thought my prescription needed changing, because the stuff I was seeing looked blurred and unreal. He charged $100 just to change my prescription. When I got my new lenses, I was still seeing the same thing. I went back to him and said the prescription must be wrong — I'm seeing the same thing, blurriness, not so clear, a fuzziness, not reality.

He checked my eyes again and said that is my prescription.

I asked him how much it changed from my last prescription of lenses.

He said, "Just a little." (He actually gave me the same prescription I had because I looked at his notes.)

I said, "What about this eye pain behind my eyes, and it twitches on top all the time."

He looked deep into my eyes and said, "You have eye allergies."

I said, "Well, that causes the pain and twitch?"

He said, **"Yes ..."**

We will call it just another misdiagnosed symptom of so-called lyme disease.

About this symptom:

You will see a blurry, somewhat unreal picture. (The unrealness is actually due to the clouded brain.) And there may be a pain deep behind your eyeball. What is happening here is that bacteria is squirming around in that stronger strand of eye

I had it for years and years. The doctors kept saying it's arthritis — nothing we can do. I believed them because I didn't understand that it could be anything else. Let me put it this way.

How many people in America have been bitten by a tick, mosquito, flea, chigger or biting fly? Millions and millions, more than you can count.

How many people in America have arthritis? The same millions and millions.

You See, I lived around the people who live in the deep woods of southeast Missouri. So let me tell you what is going on. Ninety-eight percent of these people complain of arthritis.

Stiff muscles and cracking joints — I woke up with them. Mostly 20 to 30-year-old kids have got it. I hung around them. They were my age, who live in the country, always complaining of aches, pains, no energy and nervousness. **And they live out with the sky and trees in wide open spaces where no city life bothers them** If they go to the city, they get nervous. So they get back as soon as possible to the country setting. And their only complaints are: pains, arthritis, nervousness, no energy, and one-fifth or so stutter.

I've beat my head against the wall trying to convince them that they have it and need medicine. Their excuse is, "I've been this way all my life, since I was small."

I say, "How long have you been being bit by the ticks?"

"They say, "All my life. I grew up being bit by the ticks and mosquitoes."

These people look normal like everyone else, but deep inside their brain is clouded or scrambled. They're in a very small world of their own, and they don't understand what normal is or how it feels.

The only young man that I could get to listen to me was named **Duper.** I gave him some of my medicine. (He is featured in my video.)

Anyway, they are all just like me before. I didn't believe it until I took the medicine. And now I don't want to stop taking it because I enjoy being able to use my body and brain like normal people do, without pain, a clouded brain, and have energy. It's fun to be normal. That is how you are supposed to be.

Let me tell you of these symptoms:

Arthritis — It would be anywhere in the human body. Anywhere close to a joint or tendon in either the joint or tendon area. Mine was in my hands, fingers, shoulders, neck, back and knees. But now I'm cured of arthritis pain. I've got no more pains anywhere.

The main thing that bothered me was my hands, fingers, neck and back. In my shoulder I had the classic symptoms of bursitis in my shoulder joints. I could barely lift them. When I did, there was a deep pain in the shoulder joint and ball at that time. I couldn't lift them above my head. It was a tremendous pain, a grinding sound I heard and felt.

The hands and fingers — swollen joints at knuckle area. The thick hard muscle hooked to the thumb would always cramp up with tenseness and pain. When you close your fist tightly, it is painful in the joint area and tendons hooking the joint together.

Fingers will ache with pain. I was always popping, rubbing, twisting them to get back circulation and ease stiffness. They were stiff and tense.

(In the late stage of this disease, your thumb may stick up or curl under. Your little finger may be separated from other fingers. The ring finger and the one next to it may pull in and downward with tension, while the pinky and index fingers may be separated and pointing in the opposite direction.)

The neck will be stiff, sometimes tired and tense with pain. It is bound up with stiffness. Cervical joints may always be cracking, grinding or popping. You feel a need to pop your neck, and it eases the pain, then shortly it will return.

Back pain — When you do some work, your back will

stiffen up or lock up with tenseness, a tight burning pain in the muscle. And when you move, you hear some crackling, grinding or popping. After taking some medicine, every one of these arthritis pains were gone.

About this joint cracking, grinding or popping sound, later on it's always there with movement of the joints. And when you wake up in the morning, the first joint you move starts cracking, popping and grinding. Make another move in bed, then another joint will pop with a crackling sound. Then for one-half to two hours after you get up, joints will pop and crack.

This is a very important symptom that the country people need to be aware of. This is the symptom they have and I had. It sounded like my joints were falling apart, not that much pain but a lot of sounds.

The doctors say they don't know the cause of arthritis. Well, I'm no doctor, but I'm going to tell you about the cause of and cure for many forms of arthritis.

The doctors are the ones who told me that I had arthritis was no cure. I believed them then. But now I found out that they didn't know anything about arthritis and still don't because they have probably never had it. But I had it one-half of my life. I know all about inflammation and pain of arthritis. I suffered for years and years with it, though I don't suffer any more.

Even if your arthritis comes from an injury, there is a good, good chance to be cured. Say your injury comes from a sports accident (pulled or strained muscle), from work, or from a car accident that caused pulled, strained or torn muscles and ligaments. They don't seem to ever heal, always inflamed and in pain.

Before or after the accident, you were bitten by the blood-sucking pest such as ticks, fleas and mosquitoes. The blood suckers threw up inside your system and contaminated your system with a squirming, screwing, deadly form of bacteria. Then that bacteria attacks the wounded muscle, tendon or ligament, or just gets stuck in it and thinks, "Hey, there is not much resistance in this wounded muscle. I'll just live here."

It lives there squirming and screwing around with movement inflaming, wondering, never letting the muscle have the chance to heal. Others have no accident at all and just have arthritis. It is the simpler form of arthritis. There are two ways to have arthritis. (I've had both kinds, and they are totally gone.)

People are suffering day in and day out all the time, and neither the doctors or any person realize that it can be cured. **(And if you don't believe me, all you have to do is try this medicine. What have you got to lose — nothing — but you have everything to gain. The loss of your pain and the understanding of controlling it.**

It doesn't matter if you have the accident form or the simple form. You don't know where it came from or any form of arthritis. What causes this is the squirming, screwing movement of that dangerous form of Spirochete Bacteria inflaming the muscle, tendon, ligament or joint areas of the human body. (There are no **if's, and's** or **but's** about this.) This is the major causes that the doctors don't understand. It only takes one bite from a flea, tick, mosquito or fly to cause this arthritis. The cure is simply explained by prescription and dosage in my other book. Order one or just write me. I'll gladly send you some information on what kind of medicine you need to take to get rid of your arthritis that the doctors won't tell you about.

There is only one problem about this. Here in America, you cannot walk into a drugstore or pharmacy and buy this over the counter or get it off a shelf. Not like Africa, the Philippines or Mexico. In America you need a prescription.

Their form of government knows something that ours doesn't. Just because our government doesn't allow us to live off the countryside, run open sewer ditches out on the roadway or leave dead animals along the roadway. It is looked down upon or illegal to do that, but that doesn't mean when germs, virus or bacteria attacks our body. We have to go to the educated doctors just to get a prescription so we can get a simple form of antibiotic to get better.

Our government thinks they are doing something for us, maybe keeping us from O-D-ing on antibiotics (have you ever heard of someone overdosing on antibiotics?). Now recently you have heard antibiotics are not working the way they used to, possibly creating a super germ. What this problem is, is in the form of two words — **generic drugs.**

Believe me, I know from experience. Generic drugs in the antibiotic class are not the same. The pink Squibb, Sumycin brand, doesn't come close to the effectiveness of the true yellow and orange **Danbur.** If a super germ is created, it's the F.D.A.'s fault for thinking generic could actually be the same as the best is.

Maybe those government officials in suits and ties ought to come out of their offices and visit country people who need this simple form of antibiotic medicine or start to offer mobile testing for the country people who are always bitten by the blood-sucking pests.

Spending a little money in prevention and early detection of this deadly disease before the person enters the state of arthritis or Alzheimers, and the government has to spend hundreds of times as much money taking care of them in the late stage of this dangerous disease, that millions and millions of Americans have contracted across the countryside and on vacation.

But that's the dumb, powerful government officials stuck in that building in their suits and ties, with more important things to worry about, like if they should really be letting the people in America smoke all those cigarettes that cause them to have health problems. That they have to pay millions of dollars for later health care problems or should they raise cigarette taxes to $3 a pack, trying to make some money and save people from smoking themselves to death. (Yes, it's a decision of one person may overdose on antibiotics each year while they let 400,000 people kill themselves from smoking cigarettes.). How would you compare one death with 400,000? I wonder how those government officials with all their education would compare this number. In other words, they're worried about a law that saves one person from dying where there is no law that contributes to something that causes 400,000 deaths a year. Those dummies with all that power and education. (This is no joke. It's fact. I heard it on the news about the 400,000 that die each year from smoking.)

America is the land of the free. You can smoke as many cigarettes as you like that cause numerous health problems. You are free to do that, then when you have health problems, it is time for the dumb government rules to take effect. You can't get any medicine. This is America, not like in the 3rd World. America has laws, you can't die without the government stepping in, telling you that you have to suffer and be tortured before we give you treatment. **That is our law ...**

If you have read my other books, while I'm talking about government, I have a rat story for you. Since I've always lived with the rats, rats don't scare me. I'm scared of squirrels. This story I was going to tell you later, with the story of what the government should do. But I'll tell you now. It kinda goes along with the doctor stories.

Since I've lived in condemned houses and don't have a lot of money to pay or buy gas, electricity or water, instead of picking or choosing high class friends, I'd rather pick a lower class. Some welfare receptionists (who receive welfare) get free medical treatment and medicine. So I asked them how I could get that. You know I don't have much money. I tried it, I ran out of medicine. The doctors wouldn't see me. They told me to get a job, to get some money to pay them. I said I couldn't. I had no energy, plus I couldn't remember what they would tell me to do on the job.

So I went to the county welfare agency. I told them I had Lyme Disease. I cannot do anything. She looked at me and said, "You have any kids of dependents."

"I said, "No."

She said, "You have to be 100% disabled to get walfare. You don't look like it to me."

At the time I was nervous and out of energy, with body rushes coming and going all the time. I said to myself, this is unreal. I'm not at the welfare office. She says I look perfectly healthy and says she's the one who approves the paper. I say the outside look of my body is healthy, but the inside is messed up. I can't remember anything, no energy, really nervous, no money. I need some medicine, $13 worth.

She said, "You have to be a hundred percent disabled to get welfare if you don't have any dependents. I send the paper in, but it won't be approved. So I'm sitting there, staring at her, thinking all I need is a doctor's appointment and a prescription for $13 worth of medicine. And the doctor told me to bring some money or a welfare card to pay her for the doctor's appointment before I can get a prescription for some medicine.

So I said I'm not leaving. I need help. I stare at the old country red-neck woman that works for the state government system. She said she would send the paper in, but said it wouldn't be approved. She said, "You need to go to the doctor."

I said that is what I'm here for. I already know that; I need some medicine, send me to the doctor.

She said, "You need to go to the doctor to see if you are disabled."

I told her that all I need is some medicine, then I won't be disabled. I have to take medicine for the rest of my life, or become disabled real quick instead of over a matter of time.

She said, "You don't look disabled, and no dependents. I think you had better leave.

I say, **"Leave?** I need some help, some medicine.

She says, "You better leave now. Go to the Health Department."

I told her once again that all I need is just health care. I survive without money. I can get some food from the trash behind the stores, but I cannot get medicine that way. I need a medical card.

She says, "You are not going to get it. **Leave."** Then she calls the next person in.

And I'm thinking, "You red-neck old lady. You don't understand. So I stand up, full of energy. My blood is pumping, thinking I'll just push the desk over on the red-neck bitch who works for the State. She doesn't think there is anything wrong with me.

(The story goes, she was lucky. And it was just one more time that the Lord God kept me from doing something I would regret. When I got some medicine and my mind became clear thinking again.) At the end she told me to go to S.S.I.

So I went to my welfare buddy, asking him what he knows about S.S.I. He said, "You have to be disabled to get that."

I told him, **"I am ...** I can't use my brain to think or remember or my body to move. Isn't that disabled?"

He said, "Yeah ... and they will give you money and medicine to get better."

I said, "I'm not worried about money. I need medicine."

He said, "They will give you medicine to get you better. So you don't have to go on S.S.I."

I said, "That is just what I need. Where is it?"

He said, "Cape Girardeau, 50 miles."

Let me shorten this story:

I call the office they sound encouraging, gave me a case worker. In the meantime of this two-month ordeal I went back to the Oriental doctor and got some more medicine. My case worker also told me I had to be disabled.

I said, "I am if I don't take medicine." At the time I had some medicine and I was feeling fine.

She told me to go to this doctor in Cape to see if I am disabled. I went to the doctor in hopes I would get some medicine.

I had a month supply of medicine and took it. Four days after I ran out, it was the time to go back to the doctor. (It usually takes seven to ten days before I start feeling funny after running out of medicine.) I told the doctor I just ran out of medicine, and I was still feeling good but would soon enter into an unreal state of mind and body.

Anyway, the story goes. I had to wait two weeks. They didn't approve me. Then I called the case worker three times after that, saying, "I don't want money, just medical treatment." But she says they can't help me.

This is when I got so depressed and moved to Kansas City, Missouri. I got a job there. While I was painting a black lady's house (she looks like Oprah), I noticed all these rat holes around their dog houses.

I said to her, "You got rats."

She said, "Yeah, I wish I could get rid of them. They come from across the alley at this Senior Citizen gathering place. They throw out bread for the birds and rats get it, too."

I told the black lady I need a couple of rats. I got someone I want to send them to. And I ask, "Do you care if I catch a couple of rats?"

Then she asked, "Are you going to catch them alive?"

I told her, "No ... I need some dead rats to send to this redneck lady at the S.S.I. office." (That is how the story got started about the doctor around the corner that gets people on S.S.I. and gives prescriptions out to anyone.)

But this story goes: I walked around the corner to the hardware store and said, "You have any rat traps?"

They said, "Yeah." I got two traps there and a loaf of brad at the 7-11 store. Then went back to the lady's house that looked like Oprah.

I said, "I'm back. I got traps and bait. Do you care if I catch a couple of rats?"

She said, "No ... go ahead, catch all of them."

I said, "No, I just need a couple of rats." I set the traps and the bait. Came back one hour later and had two dead rats. I went to the 7-11 store, got some zip-lock freezer storage bags and a big one-dollar envelope from the post office. Stuck the two rats in the zip-lock freezer storage bag, put the bag in the envelope, along with a note saying, *"Thanks for helping me with my lyme disease."*

I looked at the package and said to myself, "I can't do this. I may get into trouble." I took the package and threw it into a dumpster on the way home.

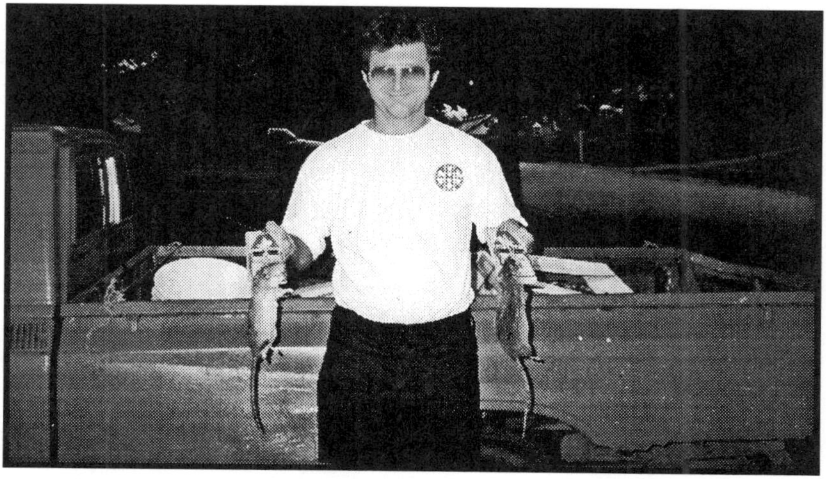

Above: These were the two dead rats.

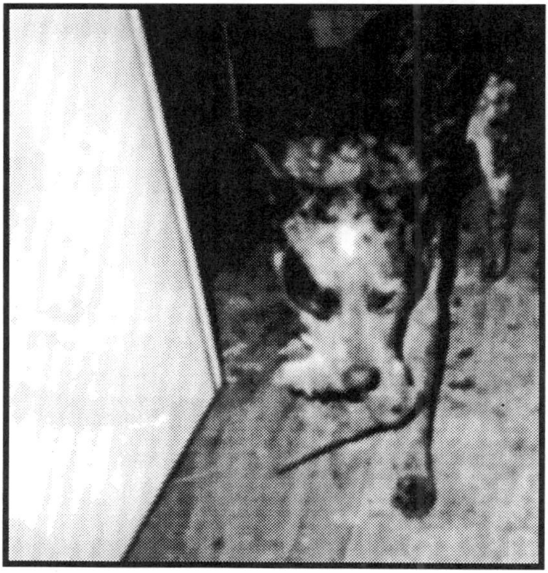

Right: My rat-catching dog with one of his catches.

The rat stories are true, along with the rat stories in my other book. See, rats and mice like me because I lived in condemned houses and throw my food scraps on the floor. It was a habit I picked up when I forgot how to spell my name, didn't know what year it was or what I ate seconds ago. This story may seem funny to you, but there is nothing funny about having these symptoms back and not being able to get medicine to treat the cause of them.

When you enter that state of mind and body knowing the medicine you need to return to the real world and can't get it, it's either time to suffer or make a joke of it. I remember at that time standing around, urinating on the floors and walls of my house, throwing food on the floor and wondering what year it was. Always thinking of how am I going to get some medicine to get better. (It sounds funny to me now, you may think I'm crazy.) But that is the way it was. Now that I have my own mind and body back, I'm ready to tell the world what happened to me and how uncaring the doctors and our government were to me.

Let me tell you how to tell if you have this disease, when you lay down to sleep at night or when waking up in the morning ...

It's a very simple way that the doctors know nothing about. If this happens to you, you are infected with this bacteria and need medicine. It doesn't matter what the disbelieving doctor says. They will not describe the symptoms the way I do because they never experienced them. They received their information from soneone else who never had experienced it at all, from a book some red-neck wrote. It's all heresay. All my information is first-hand experience. See, I'm no doctor. I don't need years of going to their school to know what I know about this disease.

See, all I know about is: The symptoms of this disease when left untreated and how the doctors, government and C.D.C. don't understand it at all. I'm like up a creek without a paddle. I don't have any money, insurance, medicine or a doctor. I'm desperately fighting this alone. No one understands this but the Lord God and the little Oriental women He gave me.

As I remind Bruce Rodgers and Ray Hartman, **the doctors' and the government story of this disease will not be like mine.** I have no medicine to fight with, whereas the doctors have all the medicine they need to fight this said disease.

The government has the power to change the prescription law to help millions that suffer from this disease and its symptoms. But they have too much power for themselves instead of giving, helping and sharing it with the people who need it, here in America.

Remember in the 3rd World countries, the doctors and the government gave the power to the people to help themselves. When they get sick and don't have money for the doctor, they just go to the drugstore and ask the registered pharmacist what kind of medicine they need. This government cares about the health of their people.

September 30, 1993. I heard on the N.B.C. National News that two men in Bryard County, Florida, were caught smuggling 1700 doses of A.Z.T. (the AIDS drug). They said, "AIDS patients with prescriptions pay $1.50 a dose, but on the black market $5 a dose. **(That is just one example of that dumb American health law. We have saying, need medical treatment with medicine, can't get it. Smuggle the medicine to the ones who need it. By-pass the doctors, F.D.A. and government's uncaring law for health care.)**

Does the government and F.D.A. understand that they are causing suffering and death and don't have the balls to change it. Hillary Clinton doesn't have any balls because she is the opposite sex. She should combine efforts with the same one who got the yeast prescription law passed for over-the-counter sales. They together would have the power, caring and understanding to change our health care system, making it useful for Americans. These women of power have a caring, nurturing, understanding, survival instinct. The guys with the balls up there don't understand. It probably comes with their maternal instinct: to love and care for as a woman and a mother.

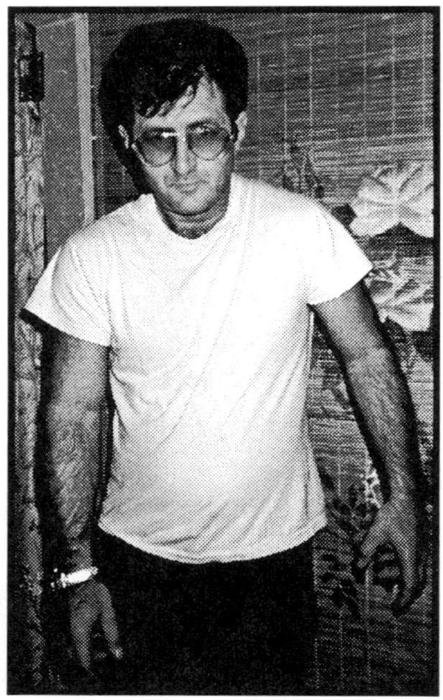

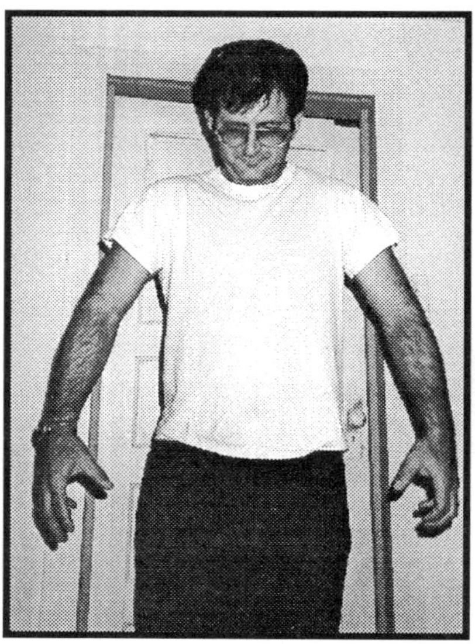

This is the tense Frankenstein look. When the women saw me coming, they knew I wasn't normal, and it would scare them. That is why I've always had trouble with women understanding me. When I'd try to talk to a girl, after the first one or two words, I couldn't think of the next word to say, and I would just space off into another world with a blank brain that had a cloud floating around in it blocking my thoughts. I always thought to myself, "How can those other guys talk to women and remember what to say?" Now I know they didn't have a disease separating the brain and body.

HOW TO TELL IF YOU HAVE IT WHEN YOU LAY DOWN TO SLEEP OR WAKE UP IN THE MORNING

Now to the people who want to understand the symptoms of this misunderstood and misdiagnosed disease. Say, you lay down, it's night and time for bed.

The first thing you will notice is, it is uneasy to relax. It seems like your body is tense and full of jittery energy. You may feel your body creeping up with a tenseness, then letting go. Tenseness creeps up — then lets go over and over with no relaxing.

- Your toes may seem to cramp up
- Stomach muscles feel tense, tight or jittery
- Shoulder or elbow tendons feel tense and won't relax
- Your neck feels tense at the back of skull
- It seems hard to relax
- Brain may be rushing fast with thoughts that pop in and pop out, then forgotten hard to go back to the same thought because of nervousness and forgetfulness
- You can hear a humming ring in your head and ears
- Then after about 5 to 30 minutes your brain goes blank
- Your body starts to relax. While doing so, your body may twitch or jerk, your arms and leg, the whole length of them from shoulder to fingers, hips to toes. One strand of muscle will jump, jerk and shake the whole limb.
- Your feet may feel like you want to stretch or flex them
- Your calf muscles feel tense or thigh muscle may twitch down to your foot, jerking your foot

Another thing that will happen is when you are laying there you feel your heart beating and blood pumping through your veins. (Feeling your heart beating or pumping is a very important sign and symptom of this disease. You should never feel your heart in your chest.)

Then when you are almost asleep or totally relaxed, your brain may start dreaming that you are falling. Then, all of a sudden, your body jerks. You wake up, eyes wide open, with a scared feeling that you were falling off a drop-off. At the same time your heart is beating real fast. Very shortly after that you are able to relax and go right to sleep. You may remember this falling, jerking and heart beating, scared feeling, or you may not. If you have a mate or somebody beside you, they will know if your body jerks before you go to sleep. This is a real symptom that the doctors have no idea of. (I took medicine for two years, ran out, and these very same symptoms soon reappeared.)

Then after you are asleep, you may not remember your dreams through the night. You may wake up in the middle of the night with your hand and forearm asleep. It's tingly and cold. This disease will put your legs, feet, arms and hands asleep with a tingly feeling. Even in the daytime when the rest of your body is awake, your limbs will fall asleep easily with a tingly feeling.

Now when you wake up in the morning, the first thing you should notice is within the first few seconds of becoming conscious, you realize that it's morning. You make a move, and the end of your extremities pop, such as your wrist, ankles or cervical vertebrae (neck bones). It will make a snap, crackle or pop sound in the joint area.

The next thing may be that your body feels real tired, such as it seems your body didn't get any rest through the night. Your body feels like it had been beaten up. Your muscles are real tired, stiff and sore. It seems like you need more sleep or rest before you are ready to get up. Your mind will slip in and out of consciousness all the time, telling your body to get up and out of bed. Your body doesn't want to move or listen to your brain.

Neck may hurt or feel stiff, sore and tired. You feel like you cannot lift your head to get out of bed. While all of this is going on, with each movement your joints are still popping or cracking. Your larger joints start cracking and popping — knees, elbow, shoulder, neck and back, when you sit up to get out of bed. Your body wants to stretch, without your brain's command. An unconscious stretching along with this stretch you may hear your cartilage snapping, feel your tendons or ligaments tense up and feel tight. Then when you get out of bed, you may get head rushes. Your body will feel real weak and tired. When you step on the floor, your ankle joints will crack and pop along with other joints. It will crack and pop for the first 5 to 45 minutes after you are up and start moving. (This joint cracking and popping is a very important symptom of this disease.) ... Your neck may feel heavy, tense and tired. It takes a long time for your energy to get started. And for you to get started doing anything, any kind of job, is hard to get started. Through the day you may have only two to three hours of energy to do something with. Then in the early evening time the neck pain and energy loss will come back. It will probably bother you until you lay down to rest or sleep. You also have to eat constantly to get more energy to make it through the day. Food gives you energy you need, but soon you run out of energy. It doesn't last too long, so you have to eat constantly. This is how to tell if you have this disease when you go to sleep and wake up. The doctors won't tell you this because they don't know it.

My knowledge of this disease comes from experience and understanding of this disease, along with the guided support of the Lord God. With this knowledge I want to tell you that one-third of the people diagnosed with Alzheimer's actually have this disease. And one-half of all people diagnosed with arthritis actually have this disease. It doesn't matter what the doctors, government or C.D.C. says.

Lose the ability to hold eye contact. When this bacteria is active inside the human body, it brings on nervous energy, and your ability to hold eye contact is lost. This is another symptom the doctors don't know about. When this bacteria is squirming around in your brain, it scrambles your brain with nervousness. It makes your eyeballs go all over. They're always moving when you are talking with someone. You want to look all over instead of at the person you are talking with. You always look above or below and look around in the sky. (I experienced this for years and never could understand why until I took the medicine.) This is another symptom that the doctors don't know about.

Memory Loss — This is a very important symptom, just as arthritis is. The end result becomes Alzheimer's. Doctors do not understand or won't accept it. They have too much education to understand this simple explanation of what causes many cases of Alzheimer's. **How many people with Alzheimer's do you think were bitten by the blood-sucking pests? Much more than likely, everyone of them or 99.9% of them.** (See the connection.)

This is how it starts out. You are in the living room, sitting there, thinking of anything. *Example:* You are thinking of going to the kitchen to take out the trash or get some water to drink or do the dishes. It could be anything. As soon as you start to get up and walk into the kitchen, all of a sudden you stop ... look around and say to yourself, "What was I going to get or what was I going to do?" You can't remember what you were going to do unless you are **normal.** It starts out once a month, twice a month, then up to four times a month. Then once a day, twice a day, three to five times a day, up to five or ten times a day. It's because this bacteria has clouded up your brain. You don't understand how anything can do that. So you think it must be normal. Well, I'm here to tell you that it is far from **normal.**

I was amazed after taking medicine. I could think of something to do. I can walk into the other room and do it or get whatever it was I was thinking of doing or getting. No more problem at all with my memory. I had this problem for years and years. Then I took this medicine and was totally amazed on how I didn't forget what I was going to do or get. I had a new brain that I could use like normal people.

Another way this happens to you is: Let's say you are working with tools such as a hammer, screwdriver, pliers, saw, etc., then you set the tool down. Seconds later you cannot remember where you laid down the tool. You **frantically** and **nervously** look all around and cannot see or find it anywhere.

So you try to think where you laid it. You know you just had it seconds ago, and it is within ten feet. This always happened to me for years and years. I took this medicine and never had this trouble again until I ran out of medicine and it would start all over once again. That is how I know it was time to take some more medicine. This is how I know that this kind of forgetfulness is a symptom of this disease. Then later it becomes more intense.

When you go somewhere, as soon as you get back you cannot remember where you went, or you are driving down the street and forget where you are going. All of a sudden, you look around and have no idea where you are. Everything looks new like you have never been in that place before. I'd get lost, not knowing where my house was or what it looked like. You don't know where to go.

Another was: I'd be with my friends and relatives one minute, and the next minute they looked like strangers and I didn't know who they were. I'd eat a full plate of food, then seconds after I'd get done I had no idea what I had eaten. I couldn't even visualize it. I forgot what words meant, how to use words to speak with. Unless you know what's going on with your body, you don't understand it and may think you are going crazy, or so-called Alzheimer's is coming to you real quick.

When this bacteria is in the soft matter of your brain, brain lining and brain stem, it will either make your brain scrambled, blank or clouded. When it's clouded and blank, all you can do is stand or sit and stare. When you look into your brain for an muscle, tendon, inflaming and wounding it. It will eventually lead to a detached retina. That is where a lot of cases of detached retinas come from. **(This cause will be found in the upcoming years.)** That is why it becomes detached. They call it old age. Why has it happened? It's because of too many tick and mosquito bites.

I lived in the country. Lots and lots of cases of detached retinas there. If you studied the doctor's appointment book, you would find that people are coming from the country with this kind of problem. Then going to the big city to get an operation for it. **(Mostly it's the country people who have this problem, not the people who live in the inner city.)**

That jittery feeling above the eyelid or below the eyelid is because that dangerous bacteria squirming around stuck against an eye nerve, causing a shakiness above or below the eye. When this happens, you may see what looks like heat or water vapor in the picture you are looking at. It happens a lot when you get up in the morning. (This is in the late stage, not early, because your body has to be full of bacteria to reach your eyes.)

Another way this could happen to get in the eye is when you chop the ticks up with your fingernails. All deep woods country people do this. It seems the to be the only way to kill them. Ticks are so strong and tough. They get the blood on their fingers and hands, then they gently wipe it off on their clothes. Then later stick their finger in their eyes or rub it on the eye without washing their hands. If you did a study on the cases of detached retinas, **what you will find is:** In every 10,000 people who come from the country the cases of detached retinas will **way outnumber** by far the city dwelling people. Per 10,000 there is a big difference.

A detached retina is dangerous. It makes you blind in the eye, unless surgically repaired. So this disease and bacteria is also making people blind.

Arthritis — Another very important symptom. Remember

answer, all you see is an empty space. There is no way of getting out or around this cloud or blank without taking the right medicine. I used to try to say three or four words, then run into the cloud or blank and get stuck in it and space off into another world. There are millions of people in the old folks homes or nursing homes that are diagnosed with this cloud or blank in their brain that are not taking any medicine at all. Just imagine if the doctors would give them the right medication to clear up that blank, clouded brain. They may very well return back to the real world. I know it is possible to return to the real world and have a chance to become normal again. I'm positive because I've been there, then returned back into the real world. So if the doctors say **no,** they're stuck in a different world, they will never return to this one, **don't listen to that doctor.** Doctors don't always know what they are talking about even with all their education.

Another short story: I was talking to a urologist and telling him about the polluted water the people in the 3rd World country drink (Philippines). I said after you boil it and let it set for 12 hours, there is a film on top of the water that you can skim off with a spoon and pick up the skim just like a piece of plastic wrap floating on the top of the water. I told him I drank four glasses of that water without boiling it and started to get a track infection. He says, "Oh no! You can't get one that way."

I said, "Yes, I did."

He said, "No, you can't."

I said, "Yes, I did."

He said, "No, you can't ... when you drink water, your kidneys filter it out."

I said, "That was polluted water."

He said, "It doesn't matter. They're not gotten that way."

So after me saying I did and him saying I didn't back and forth, I sat back and looked at this doctor, thinking whoever wrote the book he read to get his information from must not know all about the diseases they study either.

Doctors even with all their years of medical education do not know everything. And they will admit it and say, "Well, we don't know yet." **We** meaning: **We** the doctors or, in other words, **all** the doctors don't know yet. Meaning: **they** or **all** the doctors don't know or understand yet. **We** and **they** also mean the ones who taught the doctors, don't know yet either.

In other words, if these educated doctors went to the wrong school and read the wrong book, how can they understand this if they were never taught this when they received their education.

Now remember me — where my education comes from and where I got this knowledge? I got it from my own experience. It comes from not having any money or insurance and being denied medical treatment and medicine from the educated money-hungry doctor system. I learned these symptoms, question and answer from the education and schooling the doctors sent me to, by caring more about the money that I didn't have and less about the disease that I did have.

After going to this school (where I learned nothing but all about arthritis, Alzheimer's, nervousness and stuttering), I wrote the book about this disease and told all about what the doctors who say **we** or **they** don't know yet about this disease. It's because they were never taught about it. I was taught about it. Therefore, I wrote the book, and in the book I don't care about the doctors because they didn't care about me or my information. It's the people of the world who were and are being misdiagnosed and mistreated by the doctors that I care about — the ordinary people who suffer from arthritis, Alzheimer's and nervousness, thinking that there is no cure or relief for their symptoms because the educated doctors say so. **(Do you get my point?)**

In other words, even the most educated medical professional, if they went to the wrong school and read the wrong book, aren't going to give you this information like I can give it to you.

Depression — This is also a symptom of the disease. In the form of two simple words, **"I can't."** Even if you are someone who doesn't have that word in your vocabulary, this disease will bring these two simple words to your vocabulary. It's because this disease will make what used to be a very easy or very simple task for you to do become hard, difficult or impossible. Even if months ago it was very easy and simple for you to do, it will make the words **I can't** always come to your mind. When you can no longer do something that used to be done very easily, you become depressed.

This means **I can't:**

- Remember what I did
- What I was going to do
- Smile naturally
- Don't have any energy
- Do that no more or do this no more
- I get nervous
- I'm getting old
- Bend over
- Think straight, walk straight, talk straight
- Relax
- Walk up the hill, down the road, to the store
- Drive in traffic
- Get up easily, etc.,

Anything that used to be so easily done seems much harder for you to do because of these symptoms. And the words **"I can't"** cause depression. It's because when you can't do something you easily get depressed.

Stuttering — The government does not say that is a symptom of this disease. I know it because after taking medicine, the stuttering I had disappeared. When I run out of medicine, it comes back. I don't know if it is a breathing or brain stutter or if it comes from both. Brain and Breath. It can be in the form of breath. When a person sounds like they smoked too many cigarettes and are holding their breath trying to talk at the same time, or a brain stutter. Da - da - da - dog or wa - wa - wa - well. (That is another symptom the doctors don't understand about this disease). And the government says nothing about the symptom in their book.

No facial expression — When you have a blank brain, you also have a blank face. Girls always used to tell me to smile, and it seemed so difficult for me to do and so easily for other people to do. My facial muscles were tight, and my brain was blank. After taking medicine, I could naturally smile. I was amazed again, how something that was so difficult for me to do before, after taking medicine it became so easily done. I could move my face and make facial expressions. (How many people in the old folks home have a blank face, with no facial expression? Get my point?)

Talk out of the side of your mouth or mumble — This comes in the very late stage. I know a country kid, just called J.R. After drinking three to four cans of beer, one side of his mouth is closed, while the other side is half open. When he talks, he mumbles. He has been bitten by well over 7,000 ticks. He can talk okay if he doesn't drink beer. When alcohol is mixed with this disease, the symptoms come out like a flashing red light. That is why it is very difficult to tell if a red-neck has this disease. Their symptoms are more of the nervousness kind.

See, when someone with this kind of disease drinks and the alcohol mixes with it, it relaxes their nervousness. I used to drink very moderately. After two or three beers, I was really relaxed and ready for bed. I never drank too much alcohol, because it would put me to sleep. After taking some medicine for months, I tried some more alcohol one day. (Before two or three beers would put me to sleep.) I got a 12 pack, drank it, didn't feel anything. Got another 12 pack and drank it. After 24 beers I still didn't feel anything. I came to the conclusion that there was something wrong with that beer, or that medicine unblocked my energy flow and alcohol did not affect me any more. After that experience I understood why those kids who were bitten by thousands of ticks and have never taken medicine for the tick bites act the way they do. When they drank just three to four beers, they stagger, stutter, slur, slobber, look drunk as skunks, then finally go to sleep and start relaxing from their nervousness. When you mix alcohol with this disease, the effect of alcohol is doubled or tripled.

See, instead of these country kids and adults going to the doctor or buying antibiotic medicine, they use alcohol to get rid of their arthritis pain and nervousness. **They are using alcohol to cover up the symptoms instead of medicine to control their disease.** Which do you think will help them in the long run or the rest of their life? **Alcohol** or **medicine?**

Do you think the government cares about those country youth who have been bitten by the blood-sucking pests a thousand times before their 16th birthday? If the government cared about them (those country people), they would offer them easy access to medical treatment, paying just a little money now for early treatment and education, instead of waiting for those kids and adults to become alcoholics, going blind from detached retinas or just sitting in the old folks home waiting to die, where they have to pay hundreds of times more money then, just to take care of them. (But that is how our government system is.) Instead of paying 20¢ for a nut and bolt, they want to spend our tax dollars and pay $20 for the same nut and bolt. That is the way they have always done it. They have the power to do anything they want to do. They have excess money and power. Why spend it wisely when they have so much excess to waste?

If those powerful government officials wanted to understand about this disease and help the people of America and save millions and millions of dollars and millions of people at the same time, what they need to do is get mobile testing vans, go throughout the countryside, offer free testing for

the people who suffer with these symptoms (using their inaccurate blood testing system). Test them and at the same time treat their symptoms by giving them a three-month supply of antibiotics, giving them also a questionnaire asking how the medication helped or didn't help their symptoms. At the end this way would help to find out more about this disease.

What the government officials would find out is that this kind of disease is the plague of rural America, and that there are millions and millions of people exposed to this disease and they have been exposed ever since the first settlers came to settle America and that their migrating theory from the Northeast has no basis or foundation.

That is ... if these government officials are truly interested in helping these rural Americans and saving millions upon millions of dollars and at the same time extending these people's life and well being — if they care to understand this. If they don't, they will just sit back and pay the millions upon millions of dollars in latter health care, letting their people suffer throughout life with these misunderstood and misdiagnosed symptoms of this deadly mind and body crippling disease.

I have now given them the information to make the change. But will they listen? ? ?

In short, what I want you to understand about me and my book is:

- That I am a very special person with a **God**-given gift. And that gift is, since I've visited the state of arthritis, Alzheimer's, nervousness and stuttering and stayed there for months to years at a time, then returned to the real world. I now possess the ability to look at or listen to a person and can tell within seconds to minutes if they have the disease.
- The doctors are not always right when it comes to this disease or the disease of arthritis, Alzheimer's, nervousness or stuttering. And millions upon millions of people have been misdiagnosed and mistreated by the medical professionals ever

since the turn of the century and are still being misdiagnosed and mistreated in the 1990s.

- The test they use for testing for this disease in the blood is so inaccurate. There are no words to describe how inaccurate it is.

- This disease is found in the symptoms, not in the blood-testing system. **So if a doctor says you don't have it because the blood test says you don't, don't listen to that doctor. Go to a doctor who will treat your symptoms. If they go away, you had it.** And if you found this disease in the late stage, get a six-month supply of oral medicine, because it's very hard to get rid of it (and your symptoms will return).

- It only takes one bite from a blood-sucking pest to catch this disease. And that deadly mind and body crippling bacteria that was spit inside your system will continue to grow inside your system unless you take medicine. And if you wait until the late stage to take medicine, you may never get rid of this disease and will probably have to take medicine for the rest of your life in order to feel **normal** again.

- I feel I have used my knowledge that the **Lord God** has given me in good faith if I have helped you or a loved one of yours to understand how dangerous the tiny blood-sucking pests really are. If I have helped you or a loved one to control your arthritis, Alzheimer's, nervousness or stuttering, write and let me know. I'd be glad to hear from you.

"THE SQUIRRELS AND RATS STORIES" WHICH DO YOU FEAR?

I have been a survivor all my life. The stuff you take for granted I don't need to survive, such as public utilities and store-bought food. Imagine, could you live a year without electricity to run your lights, air conditioner, fans, refrigerator and T.V., or gas to run a furnace or stove, or without going to the store to buy your food or eat food from the trash. I'd bet you wouldn't even attempt it, but hey, I've done it half my life, that is nothing to me. But now ask me if I would again attempt to survive without medicine when I came across this disease called Lyme. No way. I leave the woods and go straight to the doctor and won't leave the office without a prescription for some medicien to treat the disease.

I tell them I don't want any test. I know I have it, I just want the treatment. Even though I use the least expensive medicine and possibly least effective medicine to treat this disease because of financial reasons, it still works.

If all you wanted to learn about was ticks, stop here. But if you have a fear of rats or mice, read on, because this could change your mind. Is anyone out there scared of rats and mice? Could you be fearing the wrong animals? Did you ever think about the squirrel?

Ask a survivalist if you may be fearing the wrong animal. Since I have more pages left and it's my book, I am going to share a couple more stories with you to prove I ain't no city slicker even when I lived in the city.

I have never been bitten by a mouse or rat. I may have come close, but they never bit me. On the other hand, I've been bitten by a squirrel, three different times. Now you may be scared of mice and rats and not the squirrel, but I'm scared of the squirrel and not the mice and rats. Listen to me, I am a survivalist. Mice and rats are ten times more scared of you than the squirrel is. Want to ease that fear? Read on.

Let me tell you how I got bit by squirrels. First time I was shooting one out of the top of a tree. He was falling through the limbs and grabbing at them at the same time, and he kept coming my way looking at me. I say to myself he's going to jump on me, because he was looking me right in the eye and I could tell that before he fell on the ground and died he was going to get back for shooting him. I threw the gun back up and before I could aim, it went off. The next thing I knew he was on my head and back. I threw the gun down, shook and ran at the same time. He fell off down the way, and I kept running for an additional 200 or 300 feet, stopped, and I was scared. I said to myself that he's probably waiting for me to come back and get the gun, then try to jump on me again. I waited for 20 minutes and took the long way around to get the gun.

My scalp was bleeding. I don't know if it was from claws or teeth, but I was bleeding and shaking. Finally I got to the gun and got out of there. I didn't care to look for the squirrel because I was scared of him.

The second time was three years later in Denver, Colorado, at the Rocky Mountain National Park. I was luring one over with some peanuts and he kept coming. I say to myself he will probably eat them out of my hand, so I stuck a handful of peanuts in front of his face. He comes over, grabs hold of my finger with his paws and buries his teeth dept in my finger.

My first reaction was to kick him. He flew against a tree and started climbing, got three feet up and fell back, holding on with one claw. He was wounded, stunned and half-way knocked out and looked me straight in the eye. I looked at him and said, "You prick, you are going to be supper tonight," but I was scared to go over and hit him because he bit me. So I got some big rocks and finished him off from ten feet away.

The third time the dog and I were in an open field. He was fighting with a squirrel. They were both fighting and biting each other. I walked over that way, the squirrel saw me, looked me straight in the eye, ran over, wrapped his front paws around my shin and took a bite out of my leg. By then the dog had him again. I turned around and took off running. Hey, I'm scared of those squirrels and ain't ashamed to admit it. Ask me if I'm scared of rats and mice — don't make me laugh. Remember rats and mice like me. (But now I will admit, when it's time to break the friendship between the rats and trap or poison them, I do get scared of them because when that big rat is in the trap staring at you with his big black eyes wide open, it is scary, or when it's time to poison them, I do get scared that they will find me and jump on me before they die, just like the squirrels.)

Let me tell you about the mice and rats. Well, I don't have any mice stories, but I have two rat stories. I was living in the city, in a Kansas City, Missouri, condemned house with no electricity. I bought it from the neighbor, a black neighbor. He said to be careful because there are some rats over there. I say I ain't scared of rats. I say I'll feed them and they will like me. He tells me he wouldn't feed them, he'd kill them.

I tell him, "Nah, maybe if they try to bite me I'll kill them."

He looked at me like where did you come from, and said he wouldn't even think of moving in there without killing the rats, shook his head and walked away.

Then one week later I moved in 75 chickens and two hogs right in the middle of the city (off 75th Street). Then one day I saw him with hands on his hips staring at the hogs when they were rooting in the yard making mud holes and taring up the grass. Anyway, it goes on into a long story, but at the end the animal control, which was really the dog catcher, said I had to get rid of them or he would come back and take them all to the dog pound.

About the rats though, I would hear them clawing and scratching at night, digging holes through the walls, and they would come around and pick up the food I'd throw on the floor. Then once in a while I'd see them in the daytime, but at night in the dark is when they'd stir around. They lived in the living room and kitchen. I'd keep the food in the bedroom. I'd shut the door, but it had a two-inch crack at the bottom. They'd sneak right through the bottom, come in and steal my food every night. I'd hear them raiding my potato chips, cereal and bread. I'd sleep on the floor with just a mattress and put my food on top of a foot locker two feet from my head. My mattress was twice as short as this foot locker, but they didn't get on my bed, they just went for the food. I got tired of them eating up and playing in my food, so I put it in the foot locker and would throw the scraps on the floor for them so they would leave me alone. (And we are talking rats here.) See, I was scarfing my food out of dumpsters behind grocery stores. I had boxes of old food piled in my room. The rats would get into the boxes, plus I'd throw about ten slices of bread all around the room or a half bag of potato chips, or cookies. Whatever I had extra of I'd throw on the floor for the rats, all around my bed. (Now that I sit back and think of it, I see I wasn't in my right mind. If I would have been smart, I would have thrown their food in the other room.) Then when it got dark they would come out in groups. (I mean, families of rats would come into my room and have a picnic. At this time I had Lyme Disease and didn't understand it. I was having fun in an unreal world making friends with the rats.)

Then I started eating canned goods. I didn't have any scraps, and there were a couple of litters of babies. Within three days they would start climbing on my bed at night. I'd make a little move, and they would take off. Then they would sneak up on the bed and start jumping on my sleeping bag and running across the top of my sleeping bag trying to wake me up, because they didn't have any food to eat. They did it about ten times a night for three days. It was like they were doing it just to wake me up because I quit feeding them. These were the young rats, the smaller ones of the family, probably 1/4-pound rats. (In other words, there were 1/4-pound rats jumping on my stomach in the middle of the night, and they did wake me up.)

After three days I decided I couldn't get any sleep this way with rats jumping on me. They must be hungry, so I left some scraps on the floor, and they let me alone until one morning about 4:30 a.m. I had my head on the side of the mattress. One of them came in, stood up beside my face, and I felt this cold whiskery nose on the side of my cheek. Probably he was smelling my mustache for food. As soon as I became conscious, I thought to myself that can't be the dog with that little cold whiskery nose, it must be the rat. I rolled my head over quick because I thought he was trying to bite me. He peeled out and ran under the door, and I said that is it, they are getting too close now. The next day I went and got some poison, picked up my food, poisoned their food. For the next three days I was scared that one of those half-poisoned rats was going to jump out from around a corner and attack me like the squirrels did. But three days later I was walking around picking up dead rats.

Three months later the bank foreclosed on that house, and I moved to the caves across from Bannister Mall. And I lived with the bats in an underground paradise. Well, not really a paradise. It was late winter, cold above ground, damp and warm and full of small lakes inside the cave. At nigh the bats would swoop down all around me. (But that is another story. You could say it's a bat story.) It isn't as exciting a story as when I took my high-class Aris woman friend and her three kids bear hunting in California. She and the kids were following me up the mountain exercising and I was following bear tracks, and my only weapon was a cane of mace. (Remember I mentioned in the front of the book when I was younger, strangers called me Rambo, Clint Eastwood, Charles Bronson and Crocodile Dundee, saying, "Hey, that guy is cool!")

Anyway, about them rats. I bought another condemned house and moved over there. A couple of days later these two little black boys came over and asked if I had seen the big old rats in there. I say, "Nah, I just moved in. They tell me there, there, they live under the house.

So what do I do? I start throwing food on the floors to see if they're around. It took about two weeks, and they started chewing through the floor and walls to get the food. I still wasn't scared of them, but leery because that one came so close to my face when I was sleeping that time.

I graduated from sleeping on the floor to getting a real bed that stands off the floor. So they made a hole right under my bed in the corner. They somehow started getting on the bed at night. In the middle of the night I would feel these tiny footsteps walking on the mattress. Well, not really tiny, these were one-pound old rats. I'd make a little noise, and they'd jump on the floor and run. And I'd holler "rat" to the dog, and he would try to chase them down. He knew the word rat. As soon as I'd say it, he would be looking for them. So then one night I felt these tiny footsteps on the bed. I moved a little; a short while later, I felt them again. I'd make a move, and one-half minute later I'd feel them again. **(So I say to myself, "Why ain't that rat jumping off the bed like all other rats did when I move?")**

Then after the third and fourth time I say that rat ain't getting off the bed. Maybe I had better get up. So I jump up and stumble around for the flashlight, find the light and think maybe he is in the covers, pick up the cover and didn't see him. So I pick up the pillow, and it weighs an extra pound. I thought he was in the pillowcase, so I threw it on the floor. This pillowcase had a slit in the middle instead of the end. He was trapped. The dog was just playing with the pillow, so I picked up my army boot and hit the pillow three times. Each time I would hit him, he made a noise like he was in pain, and I felt sorry for him. But I couldn't feel sorry for him because that was too close for comfort. (He crawled under my pillow, that close.) And he was still trying to get away. So I looked around for something heavier, found a window weight, dropped it on him three times, and he didn't move. I threw the pillow, rat and dog outside and went back to sleep. Well, not really sleep, I waited for daylight. After that, I poisoned those rats, too.

And that is the end of the story. If you read this story so far, this shows you, you don't have to be scared of rats and mice. It's just those squirrels that will bite you. And you can't forget about those ticks. Remember, to a tick you are **food.**

I hope this book has made you more aware of this bacteria that causes the disease Lyme's.

Every time I came across this disease, my main problem was trying to find a doctor who understood. To the people with AIDS, I would almost bet everything that this, too, was and is the main problem you come across also. (Add lack of funds to this situation, and it could be that much worse.) Could you just imagine an AIDS carrier (a prostitute, street person) with a disease that doctors don't understand or won't accept. Add a violent, non-caring personality to this, and what do you have? Someone who doesn't care who or how many they infect. Think it isn't possible? Think again.

Doctors, remember that when a germ, virus or bacteria attacks a human body and won't leave, they are going to come to you to seek treatment and medical care.

"BEAR HUNTING WITH BALLS"

Hey, it's my book. I'll make room for this story. It starts out like this:

I had this beautiful high-class Aries woman friend who had three kids. She lived in California, and always hung around the guys in the suits and ties. When they would see me with her, they would say to her privately, "Who is that guy? He looks like a bum. What are you doing hanging around him?"

She would say, "Oh! That is my friend Dennis."

Each time I'd go to visit her in California, I'd say I want to go see the giant trees or go to the woods. She was 35 years old and liked to go walking in the country with me for exercise and to clear her mind.

On the fourth visit there to California, she finally said she would take me, and we headed for Kings Canyon State Park in central eastern California. For the first 200 miles, all I saw was desert; then finally we started climbing in elevation. From what I remember, the trees were at about 6,000 feet above sea level.

We stayed in a lodge that cost $40-$60 a night and roamed around the woods. The trees were unreal, they were so big. Some had caves burnt into the trunks. After three days we left and camped down about 2,500 feet in elevation. We camped in a mountainous desert setting in a shaded campground. I read the campground sign. It said, "Bears in the area. Put your food in the bear box at night." I thought bears in the desert? "No," I never heard of that, they live in the woods, don't they?

Anyway, the story goes. I set up the tent. It was about noon and we were short on food; all we had left was peanut butter and bread. I brought some fishing supplies, but nowhere to fish.

This place was full of ground squirrels. They had holes and trails all over the place. I get this idea. I was sitting there throwing bread to the ground squirrels and think, "Can't go fishing." I got some small 1/4-inch hooks and line. I'll just put some of this bread on the hook and tie the line to a tree and catch the ground squirrels. By then it was late evening. The squirrels seemed to know what I was doing. As soon as I set the lines, they quit coming out.

So I started getting ready for the night, lit a fire and put the food in the car for the kids. They stayed in the car; I stayed in the tent. About midnight I heard our neighbor campers (three women) start screaming; then their car horn started honking, and they were screaming "bear." I look out the tent, and there is a big dark bear roaming around their picnic table, 70 feet from me. I got scared and ran to the car, woke up the kids, and we watch the bear snooping around. Then he comes over to our table 15 feet away from the car. We watch him smell around our camp, then he wanders off in the direction of the hooks I had set for the ground squirrels. I say, **"Oh, no! If he eats the bread with the hook in it that is tied to the tree, he will be pissed and come looking for me."** I heard nothing. I went over and checked on the three girls, then got back in the tent.

The next morning we left. On the way down the hill we stopped at this scenic spot that overlooked this huge rock mountain standing out on this tree-covered hilltop. I said, "You want to go up there before we go back?"

She said, "Yes … I could use some exercise."

This rock was about three miles away on the next mountain top. There was a winding road down the hill, and I could see cars passing in the valley and saw three drainage valleys carved down the mountain sides.

I said, "We will go up the center ditch way to the top."

I drove to the bottom of the valley and wasn't quite sure which ditch way to go up or stop at, and I said, "I know this one will go to the top."

So we start climbing. A mile up we came to a mountain side that recently had been burnt from fire. I didn't see this from the lookout point earlier, but knew I couldn't have been far off the trail. California mountains seem to go straight up and are four times higher than the Missouri mountains I'm used to. As we came to the top of the first mountain, the rock appeared. It was much larger but still a couple of miles away. We had to go down the back side of this smaller mountain, then up to the bigger one with the rock on it. (As we started up the larger mountain, there were patches of snow, one inch deep, every once in a while.) Shortly I started seeing bear tracks, and a chill went through my body, thinking there is a bear up here somewhere, and I'm with a city slicker woman and her three kids, and my only weapon is a large can of mace.

As we got higher up the hill, the bear trail would come and go every 400 to 500 feet up the hill. I don't know a lot about bears, but do know they probably have territory. And I was thinking this is probably the bear's mountain and he lives up by the big rock. We finally came to a point where the rock stood out, and I could see I was aiming for the middle but was on the front end of it. As we came to the mountaintop side, there were more and more bear trails. I don't think the woman and kids were scared, but I was getting scared. We sat on the mountaintop overlooking the back of the mountain facing a place that very few people have probably ever seen.

We ate lunch and walked along the bottom of the big rock (this rock was probably a half-mile long found the center drainage way) and headed downward on a different trail. We started having to jump down four or five-foot rock ledges to get to different levels. I started noticing small caves in the rocks. Then all of a sudden, I noticed this spot that looked beautiful. It looked like the place we saw that morning. It would be a simply beautiful spot to sit. I go over there and see piles of huge feces laying all over and say, "The bear lives very close to here." I was getting more scared and told the kids to stay close and be quiet.

We dropped down a couple more five-foot ledges, and the caves in the rocks got deeper. I looked around and saw this beautiful spot that looked like a front yard on a ledge that was about 50 feet long and 20 feet wide and shaded by large trees. As I looked into the cave opening crack, I saw a pile of sticks that looked like a huge nest. And I quickly say to myself that it is the bear's bed, I bet.

The entrance was just a 2-1/2-foot tall crack by 8-10 feet long. As I looked up into the bed, I saw two huge dark eyes staring at me. As soon as our eyes met, I froze with chills. I was 30 feet from the bear that was laying in his bed staring at me.

The bear started moving. I turned around and looked straight in her eyes (my Aries woman friend) and said, "Let's go now." I quickly picked up my pace down the hill leading the trail about 80 feet down. I heard this loud roar, turned around and said, "Let's go, run." Three hundred feet farther I heard another roar. About 700 feet down the trail, I stopped to catch my breath, and they said, "Slow down."

I said, "Did you hear that?"

She said, "What?"

Then I realized they didn't see or hear the bear.

So I said, "That bird ... did you hear that bird?"

She said, "No ... slow down, let's rest."

I said, "No, not yet, let's go."

As we made it down to the top of the smaller mountain, we took a rest. And I asked her if she saw the bear?

She said, "No. What bear?"

I said, "Why do you think I was hurrying down? I saw the bear laying in his bed staring at me when I said, 'Let's go.' "

As I walked fast down this two-mile hill, the farther away I got, the more relaxed I felt. Exciting or not, it's true.

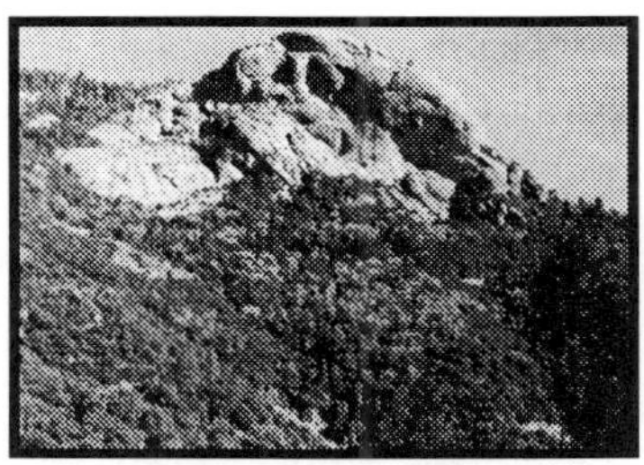

This is the rock we climbed to, and where the bear lived in California.

WHO THE MILLIONS OF PEOPLE ARE WHO HAVE THIS DISEASE AND WHERE THEY WILL BE FOUND

Can you have this disease and not know or understand it?

"Yes" ... How would that be possible?

The person doesn't understand the word "normal."
Should they grow smarter or dumber with age?
How does a child know what normal is?

Would it be possible to get this disease without exchanging bodily fluids with the blood-sucking pest?
Yes, here are two ways:

#1. Blood transfusions or donations. The government is so worried about AIDS being transmitted by blood banks. Have you ever seen the entrance to the inner city blood banks? That is where a mixed breed of uneducated, homeless drunkards or drug-addicted people go and trade in some of their blood for cash.

But what about the so-thought cleaner breed of blood that comes from the people in the country or rural Americans who donate blood? Does the government look in or check this blood for a certain kind of bacteria? Are the country people spreading what the medical world calls arthritis, Alzheimer's or nervousness without knowing it? Is it possible that these diseases can be spread this way by blood donors? (Yes, it's very possible. Does the government check for the Spirochete Bacteria in the donations of blood. "No." Should they?

What about the plumbers who play in the sewer for their

jobs. Are there any relatives of this bacteria found in the sewers? Yes, there are, and how it enters the human body of the plumbers or the ordinary person is through the use of sewer snakes, the mechanical tool used to clean our sewer clogs. This tool is dangerous in transmitting a form of deadly bacteria to the human body by using it with bare hands. The F.D.A. should immediately issue a warning with this tool at the rental stores for the user to wear leather or rubber gloves while using it (a heavy-duty pair of rubber gloves should accompany the rental of this tool).

Where are the millions of people found who have this disease?

In the state, county and privately run nursing homes (there are millions of cases here alone). **Every one of the people in these places should be checked before they are admitted. This is the place where the government needs to immediately check all residents, or the blood testing company should test the testing system here. (This is where the proof of understanding is, locked away. Once it is tapped into, the understanding will start to emerge.)**

But the doctors like to cut the tendons in the hands of the human vegetables, because of the closed fist from tension when the late stage of arthritis sets in.

This is one of the reasons they fear malpractice suits if they brought people back from vegetable to conscious human being. They wouldn't be able to use their hands because of the cut tendons.

The doctor knows that if they brought people back to this world who had lost the ability to use their hands from the doctor's negligence, the doctor would rather keep them in the vegetable state of mind and body, saying they will never return, rather than risk being sued. (Doctors have an oath and will not blame their kind for mistakes.)

Mothers, fathers, grandmothers and grandfathers are locked

away here because of disbelieving doctors who say they are in an unreal world and will never return to this world. **Twenty to forty percent of these people could be brought back to the real world, to remember their names and who you are, with the right antibiotic treatment and a cooperating doctor.**

This is one of the places where the doctors who fear malpractice suits are, so this is a tricky situation. If possible, have the blood drawn and sent away by a trusted registered nurse and results sent to you and a trusted doctor.

All arthritis doctors need to check their patients for this disease, since this is one of the biggest and most noticeable symptoms of this disease. **Forty to seventy percent of all people who have arthritis actually have this disease.** There are an estimated 40,000,000 who suffer from arthritis, and I say it would be safe to say one-half or 20,000,000 of these people actually have this disease. So here is where 20,000,000 are located, suffering needlessly from Lyme arthritis.

All doctors who deal with Alzheimer's patients need to check their patients for this disease.

All people who have lived in the country through at least one spring and summer and were bitten by one or more ticks, biting flies or lots of mosquitoes shouldbe checked. Ninety-eight percent of the old people who have lived in the country all their life have this disease and don't understand the symptoms. They just think it's old age bothering them.

Country schools need to check their children. All the children in rural American school, especially the hyperactive ones, or ones that are diagnosed as slower learners. By the time some of those rural American school children reach sixth grade, they've been bitten well over 500 times by the ticks. This is something that the city slicker government and state officials don't yet understand because they live and work in the concrete jungle, where the trees and open fields are nowhere in sight. There are at least 1,000,000 infected children that will be found here, if the state cares to understand this.

Boy Scouts and Girl Scouts need to be checked for this disease, and the older leaders of these children also, whether they are in the Scouts now or 10-20-30 years ago. Outdoor people who like to hunt, fish and camp. There are a couple million cases here easily.

The government officials who live in the big city just don't understand how the country people think. You see, the country people who were born in the country see the big city as a threat, danger and something to fear. Country people feel safe in the country with the sky, fields, trees and open spaces. These people grew up being bit by the ticks and don't understand normal. Most are old nervous red-necks who complain of their aches, pains, arthritis and memory loss.

The state officials with many rural counties need to offer mobile testing for these back woods, backward country people. They would come out in unbelievable numbers to have access to mobile testing of this disease by the state. This would also help the state to understand that there are more than they ever imagined in their state with this disease.

You see, this disease way outnumbers by far the people with AIDS. However many people who have AIDS in America, there are at least twenty times more that have so-called Lyme Disease and have had it for years and years. Remember, this disease didn't migrate from the Northeast in a matter of a few short years. It has been here ever since the blood-sucking pests were here, and where they are the disease is there also, and the name of it doesn't matter either. They have lots of names for it such as: malaria, sleeping fever, encephalitis, black water fever, Lyme Disease or DAL'S Disease. The cause is the same ... blood-sucking pests. Remember, this disease plagues rural America.

Thousands of the Third World people die every day of these diseases because of lack of money for medicine and lack of understanding to take medicine. The main carrier of this disease in these countries is mosquitoes, caused by the polluted water they are born into.

Our government has exposed millions of people to this disease alone, mainly during basic training in the armed forces.

I've heard the stories of basic training. These people are sent out in the woods, fields and swamps, the same exact places where the blood-sucking pests live. I'm sure the Big Bad Government and military personnel aren't scared of those little bitty blood-sucking pests. Maybe it's because they don't yet understand what kind of damage they can do to the human body. Maybe someone of such power disbelieves that a small blood-sucking pest can do anything to the human body. Maybe someone of such power needs more evidence or clinical proof. If that is what they need, when will they get started on it?

In the meantime, the military is still exposing the men and women who go through basic training to the blood-sucking pests, while the boss or sergeant sleeps comfortably in his mosquito-proof tent. All others lay on the ground and fight the blood-sucking pests all night long (the mosquitoes, ticks and chiggers).

What about the Vietnam veterans? Are they really suffering from just memories and flashbacks from the war? Or were they exposed to the blood-sucking pests that lived in the jungles of Vietnam? Does a blood-sucking pest have the capability of separating a human being's mind from their body? Why do they walk around like they are in a different world? Is their mind and body separated? Are they being misdiagnosed and mistreated like all the other people in America who have exchanged bodily fluids with the blood-sucking pests. Has our government turned these soldiers into hyped-up scrambled brains?

How about all the misdiagnosed and mistreated cases by the ordinary doctors? **(Any symptom I've described the person goes to the doctor for, and the doctor diagnoses it as anything other than so-called Lyme Disease or DAL's Disease. These misdiagnosed cases number in the millions.)**

And we are not counting all the misdiagnosed and mistreated cases of 10 to 100 years ago. There are uncountable millions of cases in the 1990s. Probably a hundred million or more have already died not knowing they had this disease. Remember, this disease is the plague in the rural American areas, years ago up to now. Millions contracted it in the country. They move to the city closer to the doctors (the doctors who misdiagnosed and mistreated it).

The government and the C.D.C. say there may be 200-300 thousand cases. But how wrong those city slickers are. Their estimated numbers are so far off from the actual true number. There is no way to describe how far off these numbers are. They are wrapped up in this quicker killing disease called AIDS instead of this slow-killing disease that breaks down and destroys the human mind and body. If only they would understand how to treat the symptoms and offer access to antibiotics over the counter in the pharmacy, the government, state and county officials could save hundreds of millions of dollars in the latter health care and compilations to the elderly.

If the city slickers only understood and would take the advice of a person who knows from experience, taking knowledge from someone who has been there, seen it and come back to tell about it, instead of believing inaccurate knowledge from the people who went to the wrong school and read the wrong books or an inaccurate testing system.

Remember, if you think the doctors, state and government officials or C.D.C. people know more than me, you had better find the one who lived in the fields, swamps and wood for three years without a house of shelter, electricity, gas or water utilities, or the one who needed medicine and couldn't get it because the doctor didn't believe them because they didn't have any insurance or money to get some medicine.

You show me a doctor, state or government official with this kind of knowledge about this kind of disease in this way, and I'd say they must know what they are talking about because they experienced it to understand it. But I'd bet my life you could look and look and look and never come across one. So that means they have no idea or understanding and knowledge of this disease because their education of this disease came from the wrong way to them for them to understand it correctly.

THE SYMPTOMS OF LYME DISEASE IN THE HANDS

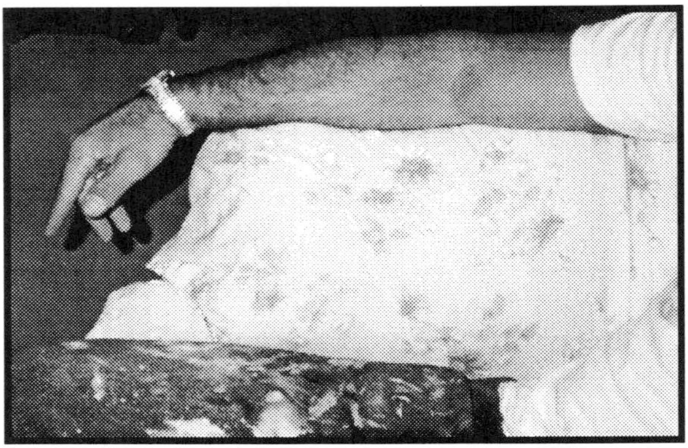

When sitting with your arm on couch arm, it feels like your index finger points downward and two middle fingers pull inward.

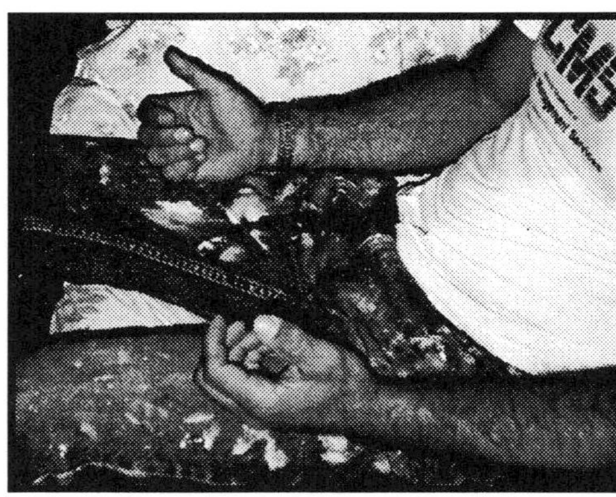

The tension here is in the thumb, fingers curl and thumb stick up with tension.

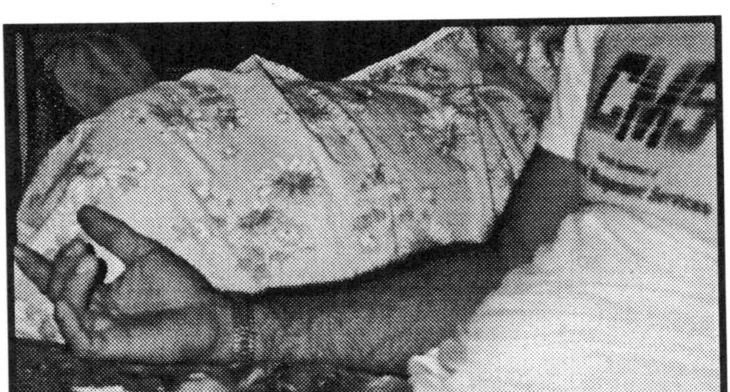

Notice how the two middle fingers curl inward with tenseness and the index and pinky pull the other direction.

ADDITIONAL INFORMATION ON SYMPTOMS TAKEN FROM MY FIRST BOOK — "LYME DISEASE: THE UNTOLD STORY

A REMINDER: I was bitten by many ticks and mosquitoes in a very short period of time. You could have one of these symptoms, and it may take years and years to reach others.

My early stage symptoms started out with pains deep and sharp in my joints and tendons. This was one of my first symptoms; this pain is deep like where the tendons attach to the bones, and sharp like you never had before.

A soreness in your jaw area, where the upper and lower connect, when you bite down or eat, stiff, sore, tired.

Stiff muscles — muscles puffed up like you have been working them hard, especially in already arthritic spots.

No energy, hard to get up in the morning, get started, need much more food for energy. (Note: a week after treatment I was jumping out of bed with an energy flow and kept going hours later.)

You're always feeling your heart beating whether you are standing, sitting or laying down. It feels like it is just below the skin and chest, not deep inside, pumping harder and tireder like thickened blood.

Blurred vision, stuff looks fuzzy and unreal, like when you talk to strangers it's like you are not really there.

Neck stiffens up, real tense, there is a tenseness that comes and goes constantly. And in these symptoms of this disease it's the body trying to tell the mind did you ever do this before. Just like the heart beating, you can be standing, sitting or laying. Say you are laying down on your back, you are slowly creeping up, creeping up, creeping up, then you relax, your body automatically relaxes, like lets go, then you start it all over again; creep up, creep up, creep up, then a relaxed feeling, then start over again, what seems like every half minute or so. It will be very noticeable to you.

Real nervous inside. I was shaking inside from my hips up, inside my chest and down my arms to my fingertips. That is why I always dropped small things — mail, paper, money, lids. Stuff would be falling out of my hands because I was shaking inside. I started dropping things twice a day, then it went to four or five times, then to 10 times a day. I told my brain that I never used to do that, stuff never fell out of my hands before. When I went to pick up small things, it would take two or three tries before I could pick it up. Anything under a pound I had trouble getting in my hands or keeping it in my hands. And it seems so simple and sounds so easy when you are not infected.

Couldn't concentrate or remember anything: a job, couldn't finish a job no matter how small it was. You forgot what you were doing, even before you got started, such as what I was going to do, what I was going to get, where I was going to go, or where did I go. I'd drive from Cape to St. Louis and couldn't remember a thing on the way; one minute Cape, the next I was in St. Louis. I said to myself that driving like that must be dangerous.

A plan — try to make a plan. I always wrote down my plans to do. I'd be lucky to get one word on a piece of paper. All I could think of or see in my brain was a blank; there was a cloud in my brain blocking and cutting off my thoughts. I couldn't finish sentences because I couldn't remember words, and I am talking simple words. I stopped at "and, it's the a," seventy-five percent of the time. It only took one small word to finish the sentence, and I couldn't think of it for a million dollars, or another million-dollar question. I would ask myself what did my body eat one minute or one hour ago. Just imagining that I would get a million dollars and I'd try for over five minutes to think of what I ate just one minute ago. For a million dollars it was only a minute ago, but I couldn't do it. There was a blank or cloud in the way. No way, I couldn't even visualize it. And it sounds so simple now. But when you are in the late stage of Lyme Disease, these simple things are so hard to do.

Three days after I started with the antibiotics, my energy flow came back. Neck stopped hurting. A week later I stopped shaking, and stuff quit falling out of my hands. It took months for my memory to return, but slowly it did.

I always asked myself at the end of a day, what did I have to eat today? It took weeks before I could even remember two things that I ate during the day. When I got better, I could even remember everything that I ate the day before, and sometimes the day before that.

Hard to control muscles in face, flush when you do anything strenuous. You can feel the side of your mouth pulling down on one corner or the other. We aren't talking 100 pounds, just three to five or 10 to 20. This one, the memory loss and knee pain were the only ones that scared me, and this one was the one I worried about most.

You can't do or finish a job, go over to do it and say what was I going to do. I don't want to do that, let's do this, go over, no let's just rest.

Time stands still, you can't judge how long it's been. A dullness sensation in head, fingers and skin, started talking with hands when couldn't talk with mouth. Stutter between four to six times on one word, any word, it just catches you. I don't know if it is a breathing or brain-caused stutter.

A good answer was, "Don't know," when asked questions. I mean I don't know about the city guy that would come across the disease, who knew how to read, write, do math. If you ask him a question, he might not say, "I don't know."

But ask the old-timers who grew up in rural America a question. If you get some "a's" and "I don't knows" or "ah, well, it's like a," they may have forgotten the word to finish the sentence. It happened to me. You always say to yourself you can't move in your brain and you feel that if you have to move you have to jump across this energy field to break or start the process. Same thing in the morning when you get up, you say to yourself it was only four to eight months ago I used to be able to do that.

One day I started talking with my hands. I don't talk with my mouth much anyway. I'm a quiet one, but one day it clicked in my head, just a click. I couldn't explain stuff, it seemed so hard. Does that sound easy to you? When you are in the late stage, it is hard to explain.

In the morning when it's time to get up, your brain is awake but blank. Your body holds its eyes shut, and you fall in and out of consciousness, and it is hard to just jump right out of bed. After the medicine, I woke up both body and brain and was right up, no hesitation.

When your face starts to have paralysis, you feel these small squigley muscle contractions around your mouth and cheek area is how it starts. Then it feels like you can't control a smile, then later on you can feel one side working and one side not on any small strenuous job or task. When I was eating, I wouldn't be able to take a fork full of food and put it straight in my mouth. I'd hit the side of my mouth and say, "s--t," I can't even hit my mouth with food any more. Also food or drink will fall out of the side of your mouth if you're not careful. I took the medicine, and the control came right back.

Head rushes, dizziness, a rush to the brain with blood, these are symptoms I always had. After taking the medicine, it didn't happen any more. It happened in the early stage.

A weakness, say if you want to move something that is light to medium in weight, you strain, get head and body rushes, it seems so heavy. I took some medicine and I could toss the same thing across the room with two fingers. Seems amazing, but true, because I remember.

You can only get so far when it comes to thinking, planning, visualizing, explaining or talking. Then it happens, a cloud or blank gets in the way, and you are stuck, you just can't seem to get around it. I can't really say how long it takes. Time seems to stand still with a dullness sensation. I say it's from seconds to minutes before you get around it. On the way around it you lose interest and jump to another thought, plan or explanation to see if it will work that way. And on the way you forget where you are going with the thought, plan or explanation.

Late stage: Your eyeballs seem to go all over. It is hard to keep them fixed unless staring at T.V. They just seem to want to go all over by themselves, in that spacey feeling they do it. When I'd sign my name, half through the last name, I'd stop because it seemed as though I forgot how to spell it. I had a neat signature before, but at the end it was scribbly.

I wasn't scared of germs and bacteria before. But now I'm leery of them, because if they invade your body and you don't have any medicine, it's hard to stop them from destroying you.

Imagine moving to this place of my own, the place of my dreams, then saying, "I'm scared of those tiny blood-sucking pests. I'd rather move back to my condemned house than to deal with these mind and body separating blood-sucking pest.

I understand the low-class people because I live with them. It's the only place I can afford where to buy a house for $2,000 and live without utilities, trash the yard and let the grass grow up to three feet tall and live with the rats. That is the way I like it (no worries). You can't do it in the rich neighborhood. There you need thousands of dollars for bills and house payments always having to keep up with the Joneses.

When I moved back into my condemned house, the neighbor on the other side (the nice one) said, "Oh, no, there goes the neighborhood," meaning I'm back, and she knows I'm going to trash the yard and not cut the grass and throw tree limbs and trash in her yard like I used to.

I had to leave the place of my dreams with my house, land, dirt, trees, rocks, chickens, turkeys, pigs, fish, etc., because the doctors wouldn't give me medicine to treat my disease, and the government wouldn't help me. And now I'm scared of the blood-sucking pests because I know exactly what kind of damage they can do to the human body. (I know it from experience.)

This disease is **real.** Believe me, don't worry about the doctors and government saying, "Well, maybe it could possibly be real or it may hurt you or it may do that, or it's only up in Connecticut, or it's only in a certain kind of tick, or it's only in one in 10,000 ticks."

They can't fool me. I know "What is real, I've been there. I don't have to wait for proof" or listen to inaccurate knowledge. My experience was real and still is. I may have to take medicine the rest of my life just to feel normal. While I'm feeling normal I'm gonna torture the doctors and government and try to help the millions of ordinary people understand this misunderstood disease with my book.

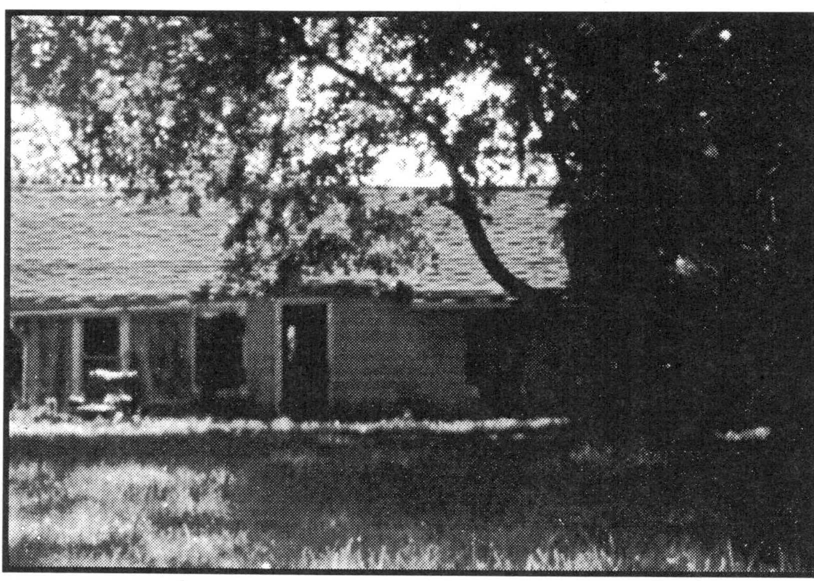

This is the house where the rat got stuck in my pillow. Five years later, it's the same house where the little spear chuckers came in and took my watermelons when I moved back to Kansas City.

THE KANSAS CITY DOCTOR TROUBLES CONTINUE

Just as in the country life with the doctors, the city life is the same. The doctors just don't understand this disease the way I do, so comes more stories of the doctors not having the knowledge and understanding of this disease, while I suffer more. They just don't seem to care or understand.

If I had access to the same kind of doctors and medicine that people with insurance do, my problem would be eased and the fight not so hard. I see people with insurance get medicine that is put directly into their blood by IV treatment. I have to swallow pills that go to my stomach that destroy good bacteria there, then finally gets to my blood, a cheap way to fight the disease, and my stomach pays the price after years of taking it.

So I go to this university hospital you always hear about it on T.V. That is where they take the people that get beat up, shot or in car accidents that don't have any insurance to pay the doctors and hospital bills. When they have insurance, they go to the Kansas side or some place else.

I got tired of being discriminated against and degraded at the inner city public health center. So I visit a real hospital that will supposedly treat anyone no matter if you are black, yellow, red or even white. It says no discrimination. When I ran out of medicine, I set up an appointment, had to wait five weeks. In the meantime. I went to a feed store in Harrisville, Missouri, down in the country and got some medicine farmers give to pigs and bees. The main ingredients were the same kind of medicine I needed and could buy it off the shelf. So what if this medicine is made for pigs and bees. I'm not prejudiced, just desperate. Directions say to mix 1/2-lb. bag with 2,000 gallons of water. I drink a gallon jug of water a day with about 1/2 teaspoon of medicine in it while I'm waiting for my doctor's appointment. After about five days I'm feeling good, ten days later with increasing the dosage to 3/4 teaspoon, I feel like Superman. My brain and body were back together with all kinds of memory and no pain. I was normal again and started thinking of all the torture the doctors put me through by not giving me medicine. I went through all that waiting and suffering, and all I had to do was walk into a feed store, pick up a 1/2-lb. package and put $5 on the counter and walk out with medicine. No appointment, no torturing, no questioning and only a $5 cost. That is the way I like it. Doctors' prescriptions — who needs them?

Soon my liver started swelling up. I got scared and started drinking regular water. Twenty days later it was time to go to the doctor. My liver swelling went down, and my brain and body started separating again just in time.

Appointment day. Time for the same old routine torture by the doctors with the same old question. So you think you have Lyme Disease? What makes you think you have Lyme Disease? Lyme Disease isn't around here, is it?

I used to live in the woods and lay on the ground. I was bitten by well over 5,000 ticks and 50,000 mosquitoes. What are the symptoms of Lyme Disease? I have all this arthritis. He says, "You need to see the arthritis doctor."

I say, "No, I have Lyme Disease."

He says, "You need to see the infectious disease doctor."

"No, I just need some medicine. I'm getting desperate."

"I can't give you any. You need to see the infectious disease doctor."

"Okay, let me see him."

"You need an appointment" (the same old run-around routine).

I say, "Does he know about Lyme Disease?"

"Oh, yes, he wouldn't be a doctor if he didn't. He knows about all diseases."

I say, "I bet I know more than he does about Lyme Disease."

He goes, "Did you read about it?"

I say, "No, I wrote the book called "Lyme Disease — The Untold Story." Just give me some medicine."

He says, "I can't do it."

I finally give in and say, "Okay, let me see the other doctor. "

"Go to the front desk and make an appointment."

I wait three more weeks, go through the same old routine of questions. At the end he says, "You have to take a test."

"I have taken them, along with 11,000 pills, and I'm not cured yet. Tell me something new or give me some I.V. medicine."

"Can't do it, got to take a test."

I say, "How accurate are the tests?"

"They're okay."

I say, "How accurate do you think they will be after taking 11,000 oral antibiotics?" On and on we argued.

Finally I got tired, shoved my book into his face and said, "Read it. You will know more about this disease. I'll be back later to get some medicine."

I set up another appointment and came back later.

I said, "Can I have some medicine?"

He said, "If you want a good doctor-patient relationship, you have to take a test."

I said, "Okay, but what if it's negative?"

He said, "We have to see."

I took the test for the eighth time. It came back negative.

He said, "Test shows you don't have it."

I stared at the doctor, he stared at me. I tell the doctor I'm 34 years old, too old to be playing games with him. He had better give me some medicine. Then finally after all the months of waiting, all the torture, all the hundreds of dollars worth of bills they sent me (which I threw in the trash), he finally gave me a four-month supply of medicine.

In the meantime, while all of this is going on, I couldn't work. I tried, but couldn't get the job done. I was living from dumpster to dumpster for food and killing squirrels in the neighborhood and finding fresh road kill for meat while the other people with money go to the store. (Remember this is my story of surviving without a doctor, money, insurance, medicine and now it's food.)

I graduated from dumpster diving for food to neighborhood squirrels, to road kill. I told my black buddy about this.

He said, "You dumb white boy, go down and get some food stamps, and you can be eating steaks."

A few days later I went down to get some food stamps. I told the government worker I had been eating out of the dumpsters and killing squirrels, even ate road kill.

She said, "Why didn't you come down here earlier to get some food stamps?"

I said, "You know I'm white, too much red tape, and they say I couldn't have then before, so I never came back, plus I can get food from the trash. My problem is medicine. I have Lyme Disease and can't get medicine easily from the trash. I need a prescription. Can I get a medical card, too?"

She said, "No, you need a family or have to be disabled."

I said, "Yeah, they told me that before, but I still need help with it."

She said, "Don't worry about food or kill animals. I'll get you some emergency food stamps. I'm glad you came down here, come back in three days."

I said, "Okay. After that I ate raisins, grapes, watermelons, mangoes and hamburgers for three months, then went back to the dumpsters after the stamps ran out.

The Operation — While talking with this doctor, he said,

"Forget about the Lyme Disease. Do you have any other problems?"

"Yes," I said. "A large knot under my jaw line around my lymph glands and deviated septum."

So I forgot about the doctor and went to set up an appointment with the E.N.T., thinking maybe I'll have the balls to get my nose and throat problem taken care of since it doesn't cost and maybe get some medicine from her instead of visiting the feed store and having to take some more of the medicine the farmers feed the pigs. (Since this is America and we are supposed to have the smartest doctors around, I shouldn't have to destroy my liver just to feel normal. They sure won't give me a liver transplant without a doctor, money or insurance. I'd rather stay with the problems of arthritis, Alzheimer's and nervousness and have a separated mind and body than risk destroying my liver again.

I met the doctor. She looked at my neck and nose and said, "We can fix that."

I said, "Yeah?"

She said, "No sweat."

I said, "What do you have to do?"

"We'll cut some of the knuckles out of your septum and slice your neck and take the knot out."

I'm staring at her thinking this is pretty quick. I don't know if I'm ready yet.

Then she said, "Do you have any other problems?"

"Yes, Lyme Disease, and I need some medicine. I know all about Lyme Disease. Four different newspapers have done stories about me, and I've written three books on it. I'm gonna be on the Oprah or Jerry Springer show sometime." I told her I'd send her some of my newspaper clippings and books to prove it, thinking maybe she would believe me and give me some medicine. So I go visit her three more times, talking on and off about the operation and Lyme Disease.

In the meantime, I tried to work once in a while doing some

painting, but it's not like when I was younger. I'm so nervous I can't get started and can only work from a couple of minutes to a couple of hours a day, then run out of energy. After that I feel like I'm going to fall over from exhaustion, then die. I just can't get the jobs done. The people seem to be forcing me to work; working is not in my blood any more; the disease took it over and destroyed my ability to work. I'll explain this later when I tell you of my S.S.I. adventures. I think maybe this doctor cares for me. She doesn't say anything about me paying her for the visits or operation. She is interested in my knowledge and my health. Before the operation I take an X-ray routine procedure and let her read my book, thinking I hope she doesn't get offended about me saying I wanted to kill the doctor's receptionist and doctors because they wouldn't give me any medicine. She wasn't through on the last visit. Before the operation we talked about the test and procedure, then came the subject of Lyme disease.

She blurted out in a loud voice saying, "Enough about Lyme Disease. Your test was negative."

That woke me up. I stared at her, she stared at me, and I got to thinking maybe this doctor was mad about me wanting to kill the doctors. When she puts me to sleep, she is going to kill me, her chance to get back at me for the other doctors. So I say to her I got another book she needs to read — it's about Lyme Disease from a mother perspective. She moved from California to Tennessee, and her kids and husband got it, and no doctor would believe them. Maybe she will believe their story. (At the end after my last visit to her she told me she was glad she met me and I taught her about Lyme Disease and she now understands more about it.) That was after the operation. The day before the operation, I was a little nervous, so I had our church minister to pray for me. After that, I know that **God** would be there with me, so whatever happened it was meant to be.

The next morning I was laying in the room next to six others ready to be operated on, knowing within minutes I'd be put to sleep, then wake up and it would all be over. Then in comes the anesthesiologist with a list of questions. I had no problem for the first five questions, then she says, "Have any other health problem?"

I said, "Yes, Lyme Disease."

Then comes the questioning. With every answer I had she looked at me with disbelief. I said I used to live in the woods and lay on the ground without a house of shelter and was bitten by well over 5,000 ticks and 50,000 mosquitoes. She stepped back to get a better look at me, then says, "Were you treated for this?"

I said, "On and off, whenever I could get some medicine. I've taken over 11,000 oral antibiotics and I'm not cured yet."

She asked, "Still taking them?"

"Yes."

"What kind?"

I tell her, and she says, "How many times a day?"

I said, "It's according to if I need to use my brain and body that day; sometimes I take one a day, sometimes four to six times."

She stepped back a little farther and said, "Where did you get the medicine?"

"The doctor gave me some, and the rest I brought back on a plane out of a 3rd World Country."

She said, "What, are you treating yourself?"

I said, "Yeah, the doctors don't understand this disease and won't give me medicine."

She left it at that and went into the next question. "Ever have trouble with your heart?"

I said, "Only when I stop taking the antibiotics I feel my heart beating inside my chest and my blood pumping through my veins."

She looked at me with disbelief and went on to the next question. "Have trouble with your lungs? Do you smoke?"

"I don't smoke, but I lived in a condemned house for six to

eight years and inhaled asbestos and lead dust all that time. And when I smell asbestos dust, my lungs don't want to inhale."

She stopped questioning, went down to the end of the bed, got in a group with a couple more interns and talked about me; then they stared at me, then left. It did ruin my mood to have them stare at me with disbelief.

After I woke up, my first thoughts were of that disbelieving anesthesiologist. Then the nurse was taking what looked like a miniature bloody Kotex off my nose and put on a clean one. Two minutes later it was full of deep red blood again. I started trying to spit bloody hockers on the floor and walls but couldn't spit too far with 10 feet of gauze up my nostril and anesthesia in my lungs. A couple of nurses gathered around and gave me Kleenex to spit in. I spit in them and would throw them in the floor. Then they gave me a trash bag to put the bloody Kleenex in and said to stop throwing them in the floor.

"As soon as you can get up and walk, you'll be able to leave, so quit making a mess." This nurse knew I wasn't the ordinary cooperating patient.

TELL THEM WHAT THEY WANT TO HEAR

It's been rough fighting the people with as much power as the government and as much education as the doctors, even though they have no idea whatsoever about this disease, on how widespread it really is, that there testing system is no good at all, that there are uncountable millions who have this disease and suffer needlessly, that medical professionals have misdiagnosed millions of these people with arthritis, Alzheimer's and nervousness who actually have this disease, or that they don't yet understand that it is not normal, safe or meant to be for a human being to exchange bodily fluids with an insect, not yet understand the consequences. Let it be that. I think I'll try the role reversal technique instead of knowing that they are the dummies. I'll play like the dummy and let them see if they can figure out what is wrong with me. It seems like a waste of my knowledge. The doctors already know me and my story. I'd have to go to a new town and find a new doctor.

You see, one of the real problems with this disease is that the doctors just don't get it. They were educated in a classroom environment, and years ago when they got their education this disease was not know of to be taught to them. What they know of it they read out of a newspaper, magazine articles or heard about it on T.V., and they just use what they think are the true guidelines to understand it, what they have heard from these news sources. See the real story of this disease is when a person thinks they know they have it, they think they have it unless they know they had or have it. Let's say "have" because it will return (unless treated immediately). See there are millions of older Americans who either grew up in rural America, are still living in the rural countryside, or left the countryside and went to the city who have this disease and have had it for many years. This disease grew up inside their bodies with them. These people can't just take medicine for three to four weeks and get rid of the disease. Neither can a person who has had this disease for over a year or two. **The symptoms are eased and seem to disappear, but when the medication is stopped the bacteria that causes the symptoms group again, re-breed and grow back. Once it is there, it is there and becomes part of your living system of bodily fluids.** Once this insect has penetrated your protective layer of skin and exchanged some of its bodily fluids with your bodily fluids, your immune system will try to fight it off, but this is deadly-looking, strong, tough, squirming, fighting, screwing bacteria. This bacteria isn't like our own that just sits, slides, covers and surrounds. This stuff screws, squirms and fights. There is a big difference. This screwing, squirming and fighting is what causes the inflamed arthritis pain, the nervousness and the swollen brain stem and brain lining, wounding the brain and causing forgetfulness or Alzheimer's symptoms. This bacteria can be controlled but not yet destroyed.

Once a person takes the medication to understand what was causing their problems, they do not want to stop because of the relaxing relief or result they get when this deadly form of bacteria is controlled. What will happen is that probably close to nine out of ten of these people who seek treatment for this disease have to go from one doctor to another doctor to another doctor and another doctor **before they even start to get treatment for this disease.** It is because they know or they think they know they have this disease, and the doctor disbelieves that this disease really exists, wanting to diagnose it as something else, believing only what he has heard from news sources or doctors' journals, in that you need a bull's eye ring, rash or positive blood test to have this disease, and wants to believe that it is only in the Connecticut area, and you need joint pain, arthritis, numbness, etc.

Since this is all they know and understand about this disease, tell them what they want to hear. If they don't get it, give them hints such as: "Oh, I went to visit my aunt and uncle in Connecticut last year and was bitten by five ticks, and two of the spots had big red rashes around them, and it seemed like a couple of weeks after that I was always in pain. Before that I never was in pain; now I'm always in pain, have arthritis in all my joints. I'm nervous all the time, feel jittery, my hands and fingers feel tingly. I always forget what I'm doing or where I went or what I did during the day, just can't remember any more. I read an article on Lyme disease, and they are the same symptoms I have. What do you think? Maybe I have Lyme disease." (At this point his response will probably be to suggest taking a test to see).

Then you should say, "How accurate are those tests?"

No matter what the answer is that they come up with, your next question should be, "Can I have some antibiotic medicine in the meantime to see how I feel and see if it helps?" This is where you need to fight, because if you walk away at this time without medicine and your test comes back negative, it will be many times harder to get medicine from them later. You won't have anything to argue with because you didn't try the medicine so you are not sure if you have it or not. Then you may wait years to go back for treatment again.

You heard my story. **If I wouldn't have tried the medicine,** I'd be living in the woods, staring at the trees, still wondering if I had it or not. Now I don't care what anyone here on earth says, there is no one who could ever convince me that I don't have this disease. No matter how many tests I take, no matter how good they say the tests are now, you would never convince me that the tests are accurate until mine would come back positive.

THE S.S.I. ADVENTURE

Do you think it is right that the doctors and state officials are always pushing me away with my problem saying, "You don't have a problem. You look healthy on the outside."

Sometimes I wish this disease was on the outside of my body. Maybe I could wash it off and get rid of it easier. Then maybe the doctors would be able to see it, then they would treat me.

I told you the story of my first adventure. They promised to help me but didn't, so almost I sent the female state worker a thank you note with two dead rats in a package. After that I moved to Kansas City, MO, went to the S.S. office and told them I wanted to appeal my case.

The state worker said, "You have to sell your land in the country first."

I said, "Why? Other people have stuff that are on S.S.I. Why do I have to sell my land?"

She said, "You could sell it later and get some money or grow some crops on it and make some money."

I said, "There isn't anything but trees, ticks and stickers down there."

She said, "Come back after you sell the land, tell us how much money you have, and we will go from there. You can't have anything to get on S.S.I."

So I'm sitting there staring at this black lady, and I'm thinking maybe I'm the wrong color because just the other day I was down at the inner city check-cashing place, trying to cash a $15 out-of-state check. I was the only white guy there, and it seemed like they were torturing me, too, because while I was waiting for them to approve my little $15 check, I saw black people getting out of Mercedes Benz, Cadillacs and Lincolns coming in and cashing government checks worth about $400 with no questions asked. One right after the other.

I proceeded to tell her the story, and before I got halfway through it, she blurted out, "You can have a vehicle. Now leave before I call the security guard."

I stood up and told her, "I'll be back."

Then I went to visit one of my black buddies and told him the story and asked how they get that money from the government and have those expensive cars.

He said, "They're in the system."

I said, "What system?"

He just said, "The system." He didn't want to explain it to me. He just said, "You are the wrong color to be going down to the 63rd Street office. You need to go down South or to the East offices where the white people go."

We just left it at that. While I'm talking about the system, I have another story.

While visiting my mom in Illinois, just east of St. Louis, I forgot to pay my phone bill. It was ready to be cut off. I remembered it when I got there. I called the phone company, and they said I could pay the bill in St. Louis at a check-cashing place. I think it was down on Eleventh Street (inner city). It was the first or second day of the month. I got to the place, and there was a line of people halfway down the block going in the place. Ninety-five to ninety-eight percent were black; actually out of 300 people I only saw four white people and I was one of them. I do admit this was in a black neighborhood, but that is where the phone company told me to go to pay the bill. Half of the people looked like drunk bums, the other half were dressed nicely. I was thinking this place is collecting a lot of money. They're going to need a Brinks truck to carry it off to the bank. After about half-hour I made it into the door where the lines branched off into three lines going to three window tellers. After about five minutes it was obvious to me these people weren't giving or paying money, they were getting money and hundreds of dollars. They all had government checks. They would hand the teller the check and use an ID or their thumb print to cash the check and get hundred-dollar bills back, not just one or two, but up to six crisp new hundred-dollar bills. It was non-stop.

I saw one guy in a wheel chair, and all the rest walked up to the window. Most of the bums looked like they had been on a 30-day drunk, ran out of money and came to get a new supply of money. This was about 4 to 4:30 p.m. Most of the women looked like they just got off work and were dressed nicely. They were getting food stamps and money back. They would hide the food stamps and put some of the money in their bra, the rest in their wallets. While I was there, I only saw one other person paying a phone bill, all the rest were getting this endless supply of money. As I walked out, the line was maybe down to 100 feet out the door. In the parking lot I saw slick-dressed black men who looked like pimps with gold rings, watches and necklaces. About five were standing around their Mercedes Benz, Lincolns and Cadillacs just waiting and talking with each other. As I got close to the corner where the parking lot was, there pulled in a new Cadillac with gold-plated door handles, windshield wipers, hubcaps and head light covers. There was a driver and three women in the back. The driver got out, opened the back door of the Cadillac. Three well dressed black women got out and went to stand in line while the driver stands by the car door and waits for them to return.

I walked across the street, went down about half a block, turned around and looked over at the check-cashing place. A lot of people were still watching me. I don't know if they thought I was a cop or just in the wrong neighborhood. I stared over at the place, thinking what a waste of government money. They must give away hundreds of thousands of dollars there.

When I returned to Kansas City, I went over to my black

friend's house and told him about all the money I saw being traded for government checks and said, "How can they do that?"

He said, "They know how to milk the system."

I said, "What do you mean?"

He said, "They have been doing that for years. That is the system."

I said, "How did those drunk bums get the money?"

He said, "They're probably on disability."

I said, "They all walked in. I only saw one guy in a wheel chair.

He said, "They're in the system. They have probably been in there for years. Don't worry about it.

I said, "I tried to get on disability, and they wouldn't give it to me.

He said, "You have to keep going back. If that doesn't work, get a lawyer."

This story is for the government, and it was very clear to me that if you want to catch these people defrauding your system, all you have to do is set up surveillance outside the inner city check-cashing places and see for yourself this unbelievable so-called milking process.

I wonder how many of these people actually have a problem as bad as mine. Possibly some of the bums do, but not those well-dressed pimps in Mercedes and those women. Remember my story, I have a disease that separates my mind from my body. I've lived with the rats, lived without public utilities, scarf my food out of the trash for years, also been denied medical treatment time after time after time, to where I'm ready to hurt the doctors just to get some medicine to treat my disease. I have a problem and I can't work. Well, I can work for about ten minutes, then my muscles get stiff, sore and tired, my heart starts pounding like it's going to explode in my chest, my energy vanishes, then it feels like I'm going to fall over and die. Other times I'm so nervous I go around in circles. With these problems it's very hard to get a job done, and the boss isn't interested in my kind of work. This disease has destroyed the inside of my body's system from the massive tick and mosquito bites. Then being denied medical treatment time after time and having no medicine to fight my disease has made me disabled. I don't care what any medical doctor says. I used to work for $75 to $150 a day; now I'm fighting for my life just to get $13 a day from our government system. Do you think I'm proud of that? So little money for a fight so hard, so I suffer more.

Then I heard an ad on T.V. Been denied disability? Call us. Call the Lawyer Referral Service.

I got a lawyer and told her I needed some help. I now had nothing left. I sold my land for almost nothing to get rid of it. The S.S.I. lady said I had to. I said, "I'm going crazy, can't get any help. I'm down to where I want to hurt the doctors or rob the pharmacist just to get some help from this disease. I'm afraid if I do that I'll need a lawyer who knows my story and will be able to help me, because I don't want to violate **God's** law or be in jail for the rest of my life. I figure the Constitution says something about life, liberty and the pursuit of happiness that all Americans are supposed to have access to, all of which has been denied to me because of lack of treatment for my disease."

So I get a lawyer and was sent to a place called Disability Determinations. A psychiatrist saw me. I told him I want to hurt the doctors. He asked why. Because I can't get any medicine.

He said, "Oh, you don't want to do that."

I said, "Yes, I do ... I need some help."

He said, "No?" I said, "Yes." He said, "No." I said, "Yes."

But then finally I said, "Okay, I don't really want to hurt them. I'm thinking what I'll do the next time is bring in a walking cane, and if the doctor won't believe me or give me medicine, I'll beat him with it for a couple of minutes and see if he wakes up and listen to me."

He said, "Oh, you don't want to do that."

I said, "You wait and see."

He said, "Go down to the university hospital."

I said, "I've been there before."

He said, "Go there again."

"I went four different times, then finally got some medicine. Now they won't give me any more."

He said, "Go back."

I said, "I did. I need your help so I can get a medical card. I don't have anything to fight with except sticks, dead rats and words. I've threatened to hurt the doctors; they don't like me. I need money, insurance or a medical card to fight with; that is because they want money and I don't have it."

Weeks later, I found out I was denied again.

Back to the university hospital. I went up there and left this book you're reading for my appointed doctor. I had to wait six weeks for an appointment. Appointment day, the intern came in and looked at me. I looked at him and thought this skinny little kid is the intern doctor. He looked like he just got out of diapers. He was so young.

I told him about all my aches and pains, then I told him to go get the real doctor. I left him my book. If he read it, he will know my story. Also I told him I want some I.V. immunoblobulun to boost my immune system. I said that is what the expert Lyme Disease doctor gives his patients who have taken antibiotics for years to boost their immune system and has good results from it.

The doctor came in, looked at the outside of my body and said, "You look fine."

I said, "Did you read my book?"

He said, "About one-third of it."

"Did you read about my troubles I have with the doctors?"

He said, "Yes, and I don't buy it."

I said, "You don't buy it? What do you mean?"

He said, "There is nothing wrong with you."

(I told myself the next time a doctor tells me that I was gonna jump on and attack him.) But this guy looked like a 40-year-old weight lifter. He looked stronger than me, so I decided not to attack him and said, "Can I have some medicine?"

He said, "I think you have had enough medicine." So we stare at each other.

I said, "I've been bitten by over 5,000 ticks. I have a disease."

He said, "I don't think so."

I said, "Where did you get your education from?"

He said, "I went to school."

I asked, "When?"

He said, "Fifteen years ago."

I said, "Lyme Disease was not heard of then, was it?"

He said, "It doesn't matter, you don't have it."

So I stare at him again and think I've waited for six weeks hoping that I'll get treated with some I.V. medicine because he will understand my troubles and story. But he didn't; all I did was wait six weeks and then get tortured again by the disbelieving doctor.

He says, "You aren't getting any more medicine. You already took enough to cure whatever was wrong with you."

I said, "No, I'm not cured."

He said, "If you have arthritis, I'll give you some anti-inflammatory medicine."

I said, "Will that cure me or just cover up my problem. That stuff won't help my brain or nervousness, will it?"

He says, "No."

He is staring at me and I'm staring at him. Then I say, "I think I'm gonna go and hang out with those crazy guys on the corner next to the mental health hospital; maybe I'll get some medicine there."

Then he wrote down something on the paper and said, "I know what you need, a psychiatrist."

I said, "I've been to three of them."

He said, "What did they say?"

"First one said I need a prescription to get some medicine because breaking into a pharmacy to get medicine was illegal and I needed a prescription to get some medicine. The second one said I needed a stronger prescription. The third one said I needed to get some medicine and help from the doctors, because I told him my next plan was to bring in a cane and beat them with it until they wake up and give me some medicine. I don't need a psychiatrist; I just need medical treatment. He said, 'No, you don't.' I got tired and said, 'Okay, I'll try this other medicine, see the psychiatrist and I'll be back.' "

He gave me an anti-inflammatory to cover up my problem.

What a well-educated doctor. So I'll suffer more, then the doctors will torture me, then I'll torture them. The story goes on and on. I hope you have learned about Lyme Disease from my book. If you're suffering from arthritis, Alzheimer's or nervousness and think you have Lyme Disease, good luck with your attempts to convince the doctors.

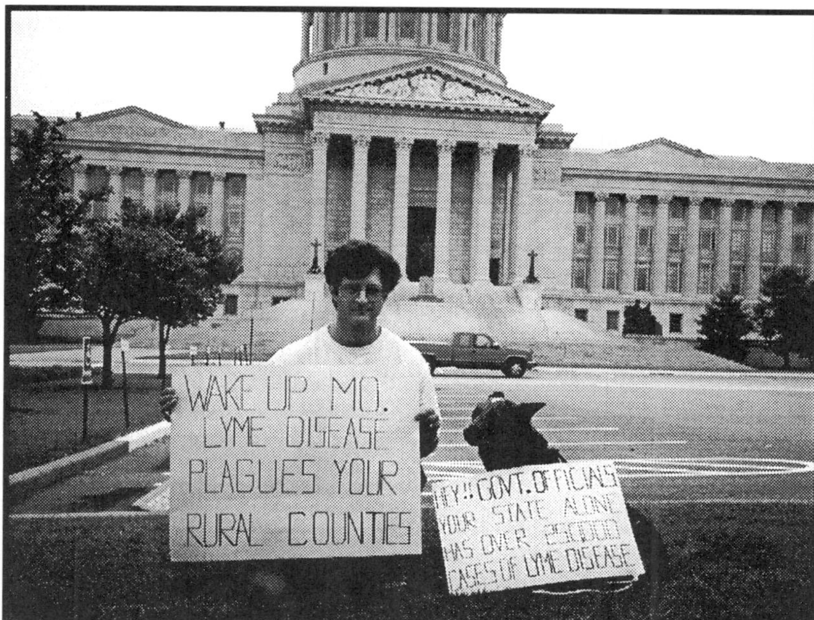
WAKE UP MO.
LYME DISEASE
PLAGUES YOUR
RURAL COUNTIES
HEY!! GOVT. OFFICIALS
YOUR STATE ALONE
HAS OVER
CASES OF LYME DISEASE

Me and the dog sitting around the state capitol building (Jefferson City, Missouri) with signs trying to warn the government officials about this disease.

THE ULTIMATE NIGHTMARE — HELD HOSTAGE IN AMERIA BY A FOREIGNER

The day the State of Missouri placed me in a mental institution for my disease — this may seem unbelievable, but it's true. Instead of the State of Missouri helping me with this newfound misunderstood disease by giving me a prescription for $13 worth of antibiotics, they sent two Kansas City policemen to my house, handcuffed me and took me to a mental institution. Me, an American citizen, and the only crime was having a newfound misunderstood disease that the doctors did not understand or want to treat. The State of Missouri locked me up for 15 days and forced me to take anti-psychotic medicine. Forced me by saying, "If you don't take the medicine, we are not letting you out of here." And what was so unreal and unbelievable about this was that this medicine called Haldol produced side effects, and the side effects were the very same symptoms I have been fighting to get rid of for the past seven years. Symptoms such as muscle twitching, muscle tension, blurred vision and the inability to think clearly, etc.

By now you know most of my story. I have no money, insurance, doctor or medicine. Only my human body which is contaminated with a deadly form of bacteria that hides somewhere in my system and is hard to detect with the diagnostic blood test currently used for the detection of this disease. I moved from my dream house on 40 acres in the country, to a poor neighborhood in Kansas City. No doctors wanted to treat me without money or insurance, and the state and county-owned health care facilities said I needed to see an expert in the field of Lyme Disease for treatment, one that charges $200 a visit and won't let you in without insurance. It's a continuous circle, which always end up in no treatment. A university hospital is always mentioned and said to be a place to go. Well, I went there, went there again and went there again. I was laughed at, talked about, had the phone hung up on me, the window shut in my face, and told nothing was wrong with me, told to go home and forget about it. They said nothing was wrong with me, there was nothing they could do, that I didn't need any more medicine, etc., so with this brain I had trouble thinking. My next plan was to walk into the doctor's office limping and carrying a walking cane, when the doctor wouldn't listen to me, or told me there is nothing wrong with me, because the outside of my body looked healthy, or that I already had taken enough medicine and didn't need anymore. I was going to start beating the doctor with a wooden cane to beat some sense in him so he would wake up and take me seriously. I found the cane, but chickened out of the plan. I went to the psychiatrist, after letting another three weeks of time go by, while this deadly form of bacteria continued to grow in my body.

It was appointment day with the psychiatrist, I went to the county health center, where it is supposed to cost $5 to see a doctor. I told them my name, the doctor's name. She looked up my name and the computer and said I would have to go to accounting to pay a back bill before I could see the doctor. She sent me there, she looked up my name and said I owed $90, which I would have to pay before seeing the doctor. I said I didn't have it. She said I would have to go back to the state-owned university hospital. I said they sent me here because they don't have a psychiatrist. She said she didn't care, that my bill was three years old, and that I should **pay or leave.** She stared at me, I stared at her.

Then I said, "I'm the guy who wants to start hurting doctors, the psychiatrist wants to talk to me. If you don't let me see her, you will be in trouble."

Then she looked into the computer and started typing

something and said, “Okay, I will let you go upstairs to see the doctor.”

By now it had been 45 minutes past my appointment time. I went upstairs to the adult medicine area, but the psychiatrist had already left and gone home for the day. It was about 4 o’clock.

The receptionist said, “Why are you late?”

I said, “They tortured me downstairs about a back bill and wouldn’t let me come up.”

Anyway, there is another psychiatrist still on duty. She set me up with him. I told him my problems. I have a disease, no money or insurance, and doctors don’t want to see or treat me. I am desperate. I’m going to start hurting doctors if they don’t listen and treat me.

He said, “That’s wrong, the way the doctors treat you. You need help, they aren’t supposed to treat you that way.”

I said, “Yeah, that is my problem, that is why I am here. Can you help me?”

He said, “Yes.”

I said that all I needed was a prescription for some antibiotics with refills. “Can you give it to me?”

He said, “No. You need to go to a physician who is a medical doctor who can write you a prescription.”

I said, “They don’t want to treat me without money or insurance.”

He said, “I can help you. I’ll set it up.”

I started thinking that this guy cares, he is going to help me. So he called downstairs, saying, “I have a man here with Lyme Disease who needs to see a physician ASAP. Can he come down now?”

The receptionist said, “Send him down.”

The psychiatrist told me, “There you go. Go down and talk with the physician.”

I said, “That was easy. Thanks.” So I go down to the adult medicine area. It was almost closing time, and there were only one or two patients left in the waiting room. I was feeling glad and happy, because I was thinking I would be getting a prescription in just a couple of minutes, and it would be easy because it was already set up.

The doctor walks out. I shake his hand and introduce myself and say, "I'm the guy the psychiatrist sent down with Lyme Disease."

He said, "You have Lyme Disease? It isn't around here, is it?"

I proceeded to tell him my story, telling him I'd been bitten by thousands of ticks and taken thousands of antibiotics.

He said, "You have chronic Lyme Disease?"

I said, "Yes."

He laughed at me, turned around, walked away and said, "We can't help you."

Then when he got about six feet away I said, "Wait a minute, Doc, what do you mean you can't help me?"

He stopped walking, turned around and said, "I'm sorry, we can't help you," and started walking back in his room.

I said again, "What do you mean you can't help me," following him down the hall into his room. **It's like he was walking away trying to avoid me.** And he was so nice when we shook hands.

Then he said, "You have taken all those antibiotics and you're not cured yet? You have chronic Lyme Disease. We don't treat chronic Lyme Disease here. You have to go somewhere else."

I stared at him, thinking what a prick he is. And I said, "The psychiatrist said you could help me."

He said, "Go tell him we can't, now leave."

So I walked away like a dog with his tail between his legs, went back up to talk with the psychiatrist and tell him what happened.

He said, "That isn't right."

I said, "I know."

He wrote something down in his notes and then didn't know what to do next. He said he would call me later. It was closing time so I left. He called back in a couple of days asking what he can do for me. I asked him to call the infectious disease doctor that I've already seen many times at the university school to convince him I need help.

He said he would call him and told me to call and set up an appointment with him. I set up the earliest appointment, but it was still six weeks away, and I was thinking another six weeks of this deadly bacteria growing inside my body. I was getting desperate because of all the pain and suffering the doctors were putting me through, and I couldn't use my brain to think with or my body to move and start thinking while waiting for another six weeks to pass. What if the doctor doesn't give me medicine this time either?

Days passed so slowly, my muscles ached, I was nervous and irritable and couldn't use my brain right to think. So I came up with another plan to ensure all this waiting would not be for nothing.

I wrote the doctor a letter myself, saying, "I went to the psychiatrist. He knows my story, and my lawyer knows my story. I need medicine. I feel like I'm being held hostage in America by the disease and the doctors. I'm tired of waiting for medicine while this bacteria continues to grow inside my body and I slip deeper and deeper into a late stage of this disease while waiting for the doctor's appointment." I said in the letter that if I didn't get medicine this time I'm going to break in the pharmacy and steal it. Then they will take me seriously. After writing the letter, I took it down to the doctor's boss, figuring the doctor's boss will tell the doctor this guy is serious and to quit denying him treatment and give him some medicine. The boss wasn't in, so I gave the letter to the secretary and told her to give it to the boss.

Two days later I got a phone call from the state psychiatrist who talks firm and slow, trying to get answers out of me.

At the end of our conversation, he said, **"The doctor is anxiously awaiting your arrival on appointment day."**

I said, "Oh yeah. Are they ready to give me some medicine?"

He said, "I think they're ready. Are you going to show up?"

I said, "What do you mean, am I gonna show up? If he's ready to give me some medicine, I will be there early."

He said, "No need to be there early, just keep your appointment."

I said, "Okay," and he said, "We will see you there. I said, "Bye," and he says "Bye-bye" and hung up.

I started to get a scared and uneasy feeling like they are going to be waiting for me to show up. The next day I was in my front yard and a tall, skinny guy with a goatee came walking up. The dogs started barking at him like they were going to bite. He stared at them, and I called them off, and he walked through the gate and said, "You Dennis Lakin?"

I said, "Yeah, who are you?"

He said, "I work for the State. Can we Talk?"

I could tell he had a pistol under his untucked shirt. He stared at me with his beady eyes. He looked just like the ex-husband of an old girlfriend of mine who she divorced because she could not trust him because he always lied and molested her children. So Knew from his looks he was not to be trusted. He was the devil in disguise. He asked to come in where we could sit down and talk. He came in and looked around with those beady little eyes and asked if I had any weapons.

I said, "I have a pistol and shotgun that are registered."

He said, "Where?"

I said, "Put up."

Then he started questioning me about the letter and asked if I am the one who wrote it.

I said, "Yeah, why?"

He said, "Why did you write it?"

I said, "I have a disease, and the doctor wouldn't give me

any medicine or believe me."

He said, "You going to carry out your threats?"

I said, "What threat?"

He said, "What you wrote in the letter."

I said, "Oh no, I'm just torturing the doctor because they tortured me."

He said, "We are taking this seriously."

I said, "Don't worry about it. I'm just torturing them because they're torturing me."

He stared at me and I stared at him. And I got the feeling that he was going to whip out his gun and take me to jail. Then he asked, "Are you going to carry out those threats?"

I said, "Oh no, I'm just kidding."

He said, "The state is taking it very seriously."

I said, "Don't worry about it. All I want is some medicine for my disease."

He said, "Okay, I'm just checking. Are you keeping your appointment?"

I said, "Yeah."

He got up and walked out. After he left, I said to myself that I don't trust that guy.

Next day which is two days before my appointment with the doctor, a white police van pulled up in front of my driveway. The dogs barked, and I came out. Two policemen were standing in the driveway and said, "Can you put the dogs up?" They asked my name and said, "We are here to pick you up."

I said, "For what?" They said about the letter.

I said, "I already talked to someone and he said not to worry about it."

They said, "We have a paper that says to pick you up. You have to come with us."

I said, "Are you arresting me?"

They said, "No, we are here to pick you up and take you to the doctor."

I said, "My appointment is not for another two days. I know

how to drive, don't worry about it. I'll be there."

They said, "We have orders to pick you up."

I said, "Okay, let me get a shirt."

They followed me to the house, and one stayed in the living room and the other followed me to the bedroom. They tell my wife they're going to take me away. She starts crying.

We walked to the driveway, stood and talked a while, and I was thinking how come they don't handcuff me, and they were **asking me** if I'm ready to go. Then I told my wife to get one of my books so I could show it to them. I picked the sentence about wanting to send a dead rat to the doctor, read it to them, and they laughed. Then I told them I have a disease and the doctors won't give me any medicine, so I may have to break into a pharmacy and steal it."

Then all of a sudden they said, **"Put down the book," like it's a weapon, and said, "Put your hands behind your back."**

I gave the book to my wife who is crying. They handcuffed me and walked me to the van. My wife asked where they were taking me.

They said, "To the police station."

I said, "What for?"

They said, "For writing a letter."

I laughed at them, they laughed at me. And we were off to the police station. On the way I said, "What are you going to do with me?"

They said, "We don't know."

I said, "I'm not a criminal, don't put me in jail with a bunch of killers and thieves."

They said they would ask the sergeant to put me in my own cell. They pulled up to the main police station. One walked over to talk to the sergeant, asking him to put me in a cell by myself. He laughed, looked at me from 40 feet away and said loudly, "What, has he got a disease or something that we have to give him his own cell?" They were laughing about it. I looked at him and smiled. They turned their back to me and talked about me for a couple of minutes, then came over and walked me to a big open bullpen area that was empty, unhandcuffed me, and told me to go in, it's all mine.

I said, "Thanks."

Ten minutes later the sergeant came over, and I asked him what did I do.

He said, "You can't be writing letters like that."

I said, "What are you going to do with me?

He said, "We're calling around, we don't know yet."

I laughed at him, and he laughed at me, then he turned around and walked away.

Two hours later they figured out where to take me, came over and said, "You're about ready to leave." They found out where I belonged and would be taking me soon.

I said, "Where is that?"

They said I was going to the doctor. I tell them my appointment is not for another two days, plus I can get there myself, so don't worry about it and just take me home.

They said, "We're going to take you to another doctor." It's about six o'clock in the evening, and I was thinking to myself the doctor's office is closed at this time, what's the deal.

He said, "They are going to evaluate you."

I said, "What is that?"

He said, "They are going to take you to the doctor to see what is wrong with you." They put me back in the police van and took me to a mental institution where crazy people belong. They brought me in still handcuffed. I sat around in the office for twenty minutes, and some guy came over and started questioning, asking me if I want to kill myself.

I said, "Why would I want to do that? Take these handcuffs off."

He said, "Before we can do that, we have to determine if you are violent or not." By now I'm tired and ready to sleep. They said that before I can be taken upstairs to let me sleep I needed to answer some questions. They asked me a bunch of stupid questions, mainly about if and why I want to kill myself.

I said, "I don't want to kill myself. I want to get better."

They said, "You are in the right place if you want to get better," and asked me to sign myself in, then took me upstairs and put me in a room with four beds. It's about ten o'clock in the evening. I lay down and start thinking finally they are going to let me talk to a psychiatrist who will listen and give me medicine. This is going to be nice, maybe this is where I belong.

I was just about asleep, and they opened the room door and said, "You have a roommate," a tall, dark-haired guy about forty years old who looked normal, just a little tense and nervous.

I said, "Hi." He said, "Hi," and I rolled over and stared at the wall. Five minutes after he lay down, I heard a quick move. He jumped up and started pacing back and forth in the room. Then he would lay down, jump back up and pace the floor again. Time after time every ten minutes the same old routine, jump up, pace, lay down, jump up, pace, lay down, all night long. I couldn't sleep thinking this guy must be crazy, and he might be a killer. All through the night I heard people laughing, talking, crying and hollering. And I started thinking maybe I'm in the wrong place.

The next morning about seven o'clock noise started, and I heard workers announce it's medication time. I heard doors banging and feet sliding down the hall. I looked out the door and saw what looked like a bunch of stiff zombies forming in line at a window counter. Then I lay back down and soon saw people pacing the hall, walking slowly and staring straight ahead, walking back and forth, the same people.

Then it was breakfast time, and I heard a lot of movement, but I wanted to stay in bed. After about forty-five minutes they told me to come and eat. I ate, checked out everybody and went back to the room. There were about five people that kept walking back and forth down the hall. They could barely pick their feet off the ground, and they moved six to eight inches at a time, real slow like zombies. I was thinking they looked like they were on some heavy drugs, all downed out, but their eyes were wide open. I stayed in the room all day; my roommate kept walking in and out of the room. That night he started the same old routine again. He lay down two minutes, sat up and walked around and stared at the window, lay down two minutes and got up and walked around for eight minutes constantly non-stop. I was thinking how does this guy get any sleep.

About midnight they brought in another guy. He smelled like a bum off the street. He was tall, skinny and stunk like he hadn't changed his clothes in months. He lay down; five minutes later he burst out laughing real loud for over a minute, just laughing to himself. I woke up scared, thinking this guy must be crazy. Abut every ten minutes he burst out laughing real loud. The old woman across the hall would be crying. It went on all night long non-stop until about three in the morning. I couldn't get any sleep thinking there was no telling what these crazy people would do to me if I fell asleep. I had better stay awake. So all night long the one nervous guy paced the floor of our little room while the other guy burst out laughing and the old lady across the hall would cry. I thought, man, I'm going to go crazy in here. I told myself, where is that doctor I'm supposed to talk to so I can get out of here.

The next morning same old routine noises started. They announced medication time. Doors opened, and a bunch of people slid their feet down the hall and lined up at the window. I went down to check it out and saw they were giving out pills with a glass of water. They put a pill in their mouth and took a drink of water, then went back to the room. I figured this was what turns them into stiff zombies. I went back to the room.

Later a woman psychologist talked with me, saying the psychiatrist doctor would talk to me later that day, along with a group of psychologists. But in the meantime, they had some medicine for me.

I said, "What kind?"

She said, "It will just help you to sleep."

I said, "I need something to keep me awake."

She said, "It's there if you need it," saying she will come back to get me when it's time to see the doctor. I was thinking finally I would get to talk with a doctor who would listen. They brought me in and said, "Sit down." There were five people sitting in a half circle. They introduced themselves, one psychiatrist and four psychologists. The psychiatrist doctor is from India. He was a foreigner who barely spoke understandable English. They all looked at me and I looked at them.

Then the doctor says, "Toe, vot is or probm?"

I said, "Huh?"

Then one of the psychologists said, "Why are you here?"

I said, "The police brought me here."

They said, "Why?"

I said, "I don't know."

The doctor said, "Toe, vot about T lette?"

I say, "Huh?"

One of the psychologists said, "What about this letter. Did you write it?"

I said, "Yeah..."

The other psychologist said, "How come?"

I said, "The dumb doctor won't listen to me or give me any medicine."

Doc says, "O well, giv oh medeson. Tell E aboot tis dises yo have I no nuthing aboot it."

I say, "Huh?"

The other psychologist says, "How do you know you have Lyme Disease? Your tests were negative."

I said, "I have forty acres of land, lived in the woods and laid on the ground through winter, spring, summer, fall months without a house of shelter or public utilities. I was bitten by thousands of ticks during this time and caught a disease the doctors don't understand about and won't give me any medicine."

By now the doctor tried to talk clear and said, "I don't believe you saying I don't believe anything you said."

I said, "Huh?"

He said, "You did not own any land or lived in the woods."

"I said, "What?"

He said, "I don't believe you."

I stared at him, he stared at me. The four other so-called doctors stared at me, and no one said anything. I was thinking to myself, Oh, no! These doctors are going to give me trouble, too.

Then he says, "I tink ou imagin it."

I say, "Huh?" Then it starts all over again.

The psychologist in the first chair says, "Could you just be imagining it."

I said, "Imagining what?"

The next psychologist in line said, "You may imagine or dreamed this thing up and there is nothing wrong with you."

I screamed out, "Ain't you dummies listening to me? I thought you were smart doctors that are supposed to listen to and help me."

The third psychologist in line said, "We are going to help you. I heard you wrote a book."

"Yes, I wrote a book to tell the world my story and my trouble with this disease and about the uncaring, disbelieving, money-hungry doctors." And then I said, "You know what I plan to do next?"

One of them softly said, "What?"

I said, "Next time I go to the doctor and try to get some medicine for my disease I'm going to bring in a walking cane and when they start questioning me with disbelief and say nothing is wrong with me, I'm going to beat them with my cane until they wake up or listen to me."

Every one of those so-called doctors straightened up in their chairs at the same time and started listening to me.

One said, "Tell me more. Do you want to kill yourself?"

I said, "Kill myself, what for? I want to get better."

Then one said, "Do you ever have people talking to you that are not there?"

I said, "No."

The other said, "Do you ever see things that are not there?"

I said, "No."

The psychiatrist said, "Tel me aboot tis dises? Ou tink ou no mor T MD do?"

I said, "Huh?"

The next psychologist says, "What makes you think you are smarter than the doctors?"

I said, "I've been bitten by ticks and they haven't. I know the symptoms and said, "What do you know about this disease?"

He said, "Nothing — you tell me." He asked about my symptoms, and I told him. Then he said, 'You need to take your medicine."

I said, "I don't have any."

He said, **"We have some for you."**

And I say, "What? That stuff that makes them walk up and down the hall slowly moving six to eight inches at a time dragging their feet? No, Doc, I need something to give me energy. I don't need to be downed out."

He said, "Ou hav to tek tis medsin so we can evaluate you."

I said, "No, Doc, I need energy. It's either antibiotics or speed."

Then they said, "Time is up. You can leave and don't forget to take your medicine."

Later that evening they announced medication time. Everybody slid their feet down the hall and lined up. I went down and stood around and watched them take medicine and saw the old lady that cried at night didn't want to take hers. They put it in her hand, and she put it down on the table top. They put it back in her hand, she set it down and said, "No, I don't want it.

They said, "The doctor said you have to take it."

She said, "No, I don't want it. I'm not going to take it — it makes me stutter and be nervous. I don't want it any more." Then she walked away. They wrote something down, and that was it.

Later that night about eleven o'clock I heard some doors

open and heard the old lady screaming, "No, I don't want to take it," and she's crying, saying, "No, no, no!"

They said, "The doctor said you need this medicine, and if you don't take it, it will be harder for you."

She is screaming and crying no, no, no.

They said, "Come with us." She is crying and screaming. I looked out and saw three big muscle-bound 250-pound guys and two females holding her down on the floor. She is still screaming, "It's not fair, it's not fair."

They told her to relax, but she kept fighting and crying.

They said, "The doctor said you need this, now relax." They gave her a shot, and all the screaming was over. She was shaking and crying as they walked her back to the room, and she was so weak and hoarse from screaming she can barely speak, but she was still saying, "It's not fair, it's not fair."

They took her to the room, and for the next fifteen minutes she continued to cry and say it's not fair, it's not fair. Then she went to sleep, and I was thinking **Damn, what a trip.** I hoped they wouldn't do that to me because I wasn't taking their medication that they want me to.

The next morning the same old routine — medication time, everybody lined up. The line was straighter and bigger, but I wasn't ready to take any of their medicine yet, so I asked some guy what does that medicine do to you? He said it makes you relax.

I said, "Oh yeah, is that why everybody walks like zombies?"

He said, "Yeah, you should try it."

So that evening I stood in line to get me some. The distributor handed me some medicine and a cup of water and gave me a big smile like **finally you're going to join the crowd.** After taking the medicine, forty-five minutes later I felt relaxed. But a couple of hours later I was all tense, jittery, I could not sleep, and my legs kept twitching.

Next morning I lined up and took some more. Forty-five

minutes later I was relaxed. Hours later I was tense, jittery, I could not sit still, and my leg twitched.

So I told the distributor that this medicine made my body feel like this. She said that those are the side effects of the medicine.

I said, "No, I don't want it any more."

She said, "The doctor says you need to take it."

So I think back to the old lady and what they did to her and said to myself that maybe I had better take it. I took it and went back to the room. Hours later the side effects hit me. I was tense, nervous, jittery, stiff, and I couldn't read or think to make any sense. I said to myself that I would not take any more medicine and told the doctor I didn't want any more medicine because it makes the same symptoms of Lyme Disease — the disease that I'm fighting to get rid of.

He said, "We need to evaluate you. You need that medicine."

I said, "No, Doc, I want to go home."

He said, "No, we need to find out what's wrong with you first."

I said, "I know what is wrong with me. I've been bitten by too many ticks and mosquitoes. I have a disease inside my body. I need a different kind of medicine from what you have. I need an antibiotic; the stuff you have is not good for me, just let me go home. I'm going to go crazy in this place. I'll get medicine from some place else. I don't need any more help. Matter of fact, I don't need any more medicine, I'm cured. Let me out of here so I can go home."

He said, "No, you can't leave yet. You have to take medication."

It was like this foreigner who was a doctor was holding me hostage in America. I was trying to be as nice as I could to him, while I figured out how to escape, and I was thinking how can this happen in America? This was unreal like a nightmare that I couldn't get away or wake up from. So I figured it was time to make a new plan because this dumb doctor who admitted to me he knew nothing about Lyme Disease has just got me by the balls and wouldn't let go. So I tried to use my brain for a new plan and find out I could not think, concentrate, visualize or remember because of taking this medicine, mixed with the fact that I have Lyme disease. The only thing that seemed to come up in my thoughts was that **I needed to stop taking this anti-psychotic drug so I could use my brain to think again.**

I remember stories on TV where people would put the medicine that they didn't want to take under their tongue. So I said to myself that I would try that. Next time they called medication time I lined up nervously, held my tongue up, threw it in right under my tongue. I took a drink and walked away, thinking, "Yes, I did it." I went to the drinking fountain, took a few more drinks as if to wash it down, then went to the restroom and spit it out. Next line-up I did it again. Third time I did it again. Then I was able to use my brain again, so I told the doctor I took the medicine and that I feel good and was ready to go home.

He said, "No, you have to take a test. And one of the psychologists thinks you need a cat scan of your brain before you can leave."

I said, "I don't need a cat scan, my brain is fine; that medicine is working." I noticed he always asked other people there, "Do you think the medicine is working? Do you think you are ready to go home?" If they say no, they will stay longer. If they say yes, they get out in one or two days.

I thought that would be the plan ... just tell him I'm ready, and a couple of days later I could leave. All the patients are always saying, "I think I'm ready to go home." So I figured instead of saying I think I'm ready, I would say I know I'm ready to leave. It would be much more positive sounding.

It was medication line-up again, and the distributor was a new person, an old lady. She was watching everyone taking their medication. I nervously threw it in my mouth, and it landed on top of my tongue. I could not move it around, so I had to swallow it. That night the side effects of the medicine hit me. I was irritable, stiff and tense all night long. The next morning the same old lady is watching people take medicine again. I was nervous, and it lands on the top of my tongue. I think, "Oh, no! I have to swallow it again. A couple of hours later, I was so irritable and nervous, I could not stand it. It was like I was going crazy with nervousness. Then the psychologist came in and said, "Are you ready for your test?"

I was thinking that I'm nervous, can't concentrate or read. And I have to sit down and take a 400-question test, and it's supposed to take three to five hours. I didn't think I could do it, but I agreed to take it because this is what I had been waiting for, and the doctor says I have to take it before I can go home. This was really the ultimate nightmare, because the hardest things for me to do even when I am normal is to read, spell and comprehend. I thought if I failed the test I might never leave. I passed the put-the-square-peg-in-the-square-hole test and the round-peg-in-the-round-hole test and some more easy ones. Then the 400-question test — it was one of the hardest things I have ever done in my life. They were easy questions; what made them so hard was the medicine they gave me blocked my ability to think clearly, comprehend and made me nervous, in this state of mind and body having to read a 400-question test that was designed to get harder with each question.

My brain was ready to explode and my body was ready to jump out of my skin. After the test I was totally drained of energy; all I wanted to do was sleep and think of nothing. I continued to act like I was taking the medicine, and I figured out how to hide it by throwing it in my mouth real quick and covering my mouth with my hands at the same time. That way they could not tell if my tongue was up or down. Then I walked in the bathroom and spit it out.

It had been a week, and I was getting depressed and asked how I did on the test. He'd give excuses that it wasn't graded yet, then he would give the excuse that I needed to take more medicine to see if it's working before they let me go. Then the excuse was I needed a cat scan to check my brain. I told him I knew I was ready to leave and the medicine is working fine.

He'd look at me and say, "I'm not done with you yet," or "No, I don't think you are ready to leave yet."

Then I asked about signing myself out, and they said after I do that they can keep me up to seventy-two hours. And if they don't let me go, they will take me to the court in front of a judge to hold me any longer and can hold me for another twenty-one days up to a hundred and twenty days.

Now more and more I said, "When can I go home? When can I get out of here? I don't belong here. Let me out, let me go home. I'm going crazy in here."

He'd say, "We're not done with you yet," or "I don't think you are ready."

At the end, one of the psychologists told me I could get a lawyer to represent me in court if they try to hold me any longer.

I said, "Why didn't you tell me that before?"

So I signed another paper that is for my release. And the foreign doctor had seventy-two hours to decide if I still needed to stay or could go. I obtained a lawyer and waited for the whole seventy-two hours.

The psychiatrist said, "I want to keep you for another twenty-one days to see what is wrong with you and if the medicine is working good."

By now I was tired of kissing this doctor's behind who knew nothing about Lyme Disease and couldn't speak understandable English. I made friends with one of the psychologists, and she said she would help me get out. She was the one who told me the doctor didn't know about Lyme Disease and was learning all about it from me.

Fifteen days after this unbelievable ordeal started, they took me to court with my lawyer. It was thrown out. The court documents revealed that I was charged with ... this was taken from the court documents as said.

IN THE CIRCUIT COURT OF
____________COUNTY OF MISSOURI
PROBATE DIVISION
In the matter of LAKIN, DENNIS, respondent,
a person alleged to be mentally ill.
PETITION FOR INVOLUNTARY DETENTION AND TREATMENT

That the respondent has a mental illness, and by reason of such mental illness, continues to present a likelihood of serious physical harm to himself or other and is in need of continued detention and treatment for such mental illness for a period not to exceed 21 days.

The facts that substantiate the petitioner's belief that the respondent is mentally ill are: This patient has a diagnosis of Delusional Disorder. Mixed Type (Grandiose, persecutory, somatic). He says that he has Lyme's Disease and that the doctors do not believe him (has had 6 negative tests for Lyme's Disease) and that they (the doctors) are not as educated as he is regarding Lyme's Disease.

Upon my release from the mental institution, the psychologist asked me what they can do to help me.

I said, "Help me find a doctor who believes in Lyme Disease and who will listen to me and give me medicine."

She wrote my request down, then said, "You are free to go," and that was it. I was glad to be free. I learned my lesson about torturing the doctor, but still the fact is I have chronic Lyme Disease and no doctor who will help me. This will always be a never ending story. I hope you learned from and enjoyed my book.

— THE END FOR NOW —

DAL

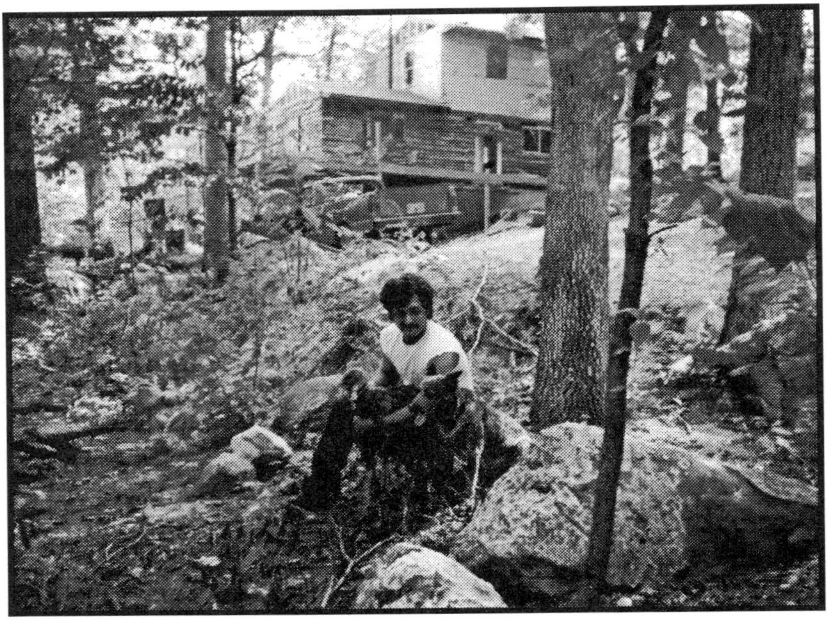

This was the house I finally built in the country, right in the middle of my 40 acres.

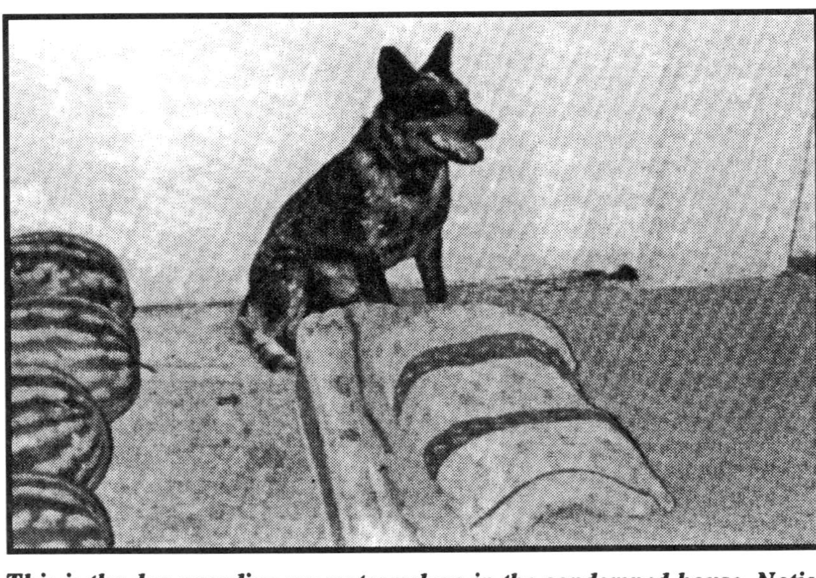

This is the dog guarding my watermelons in the condemned house. Notice the rat hole in the right corner and how close my bed on the floor was to it.

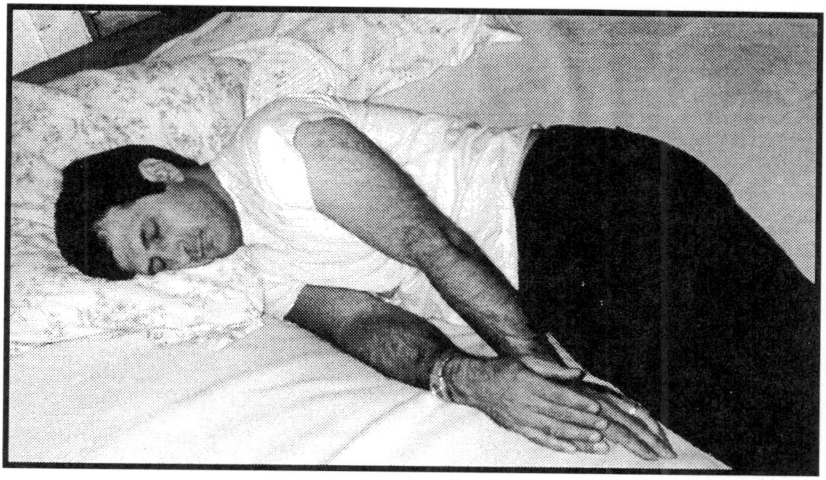

This is how I had to sleep to keep my hands from falling asleep at night with arms in a straight position.

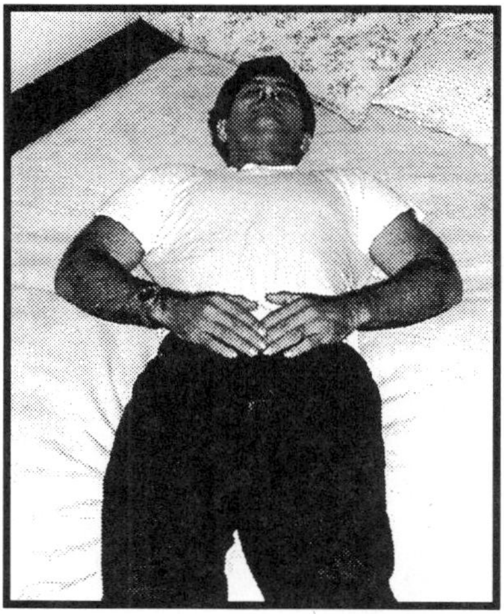

When my hands would be anywhere above my belly bottom, within minutes they would get numb and tingly. After taking the medication, this problem I had for over 10 years instantly vanished.

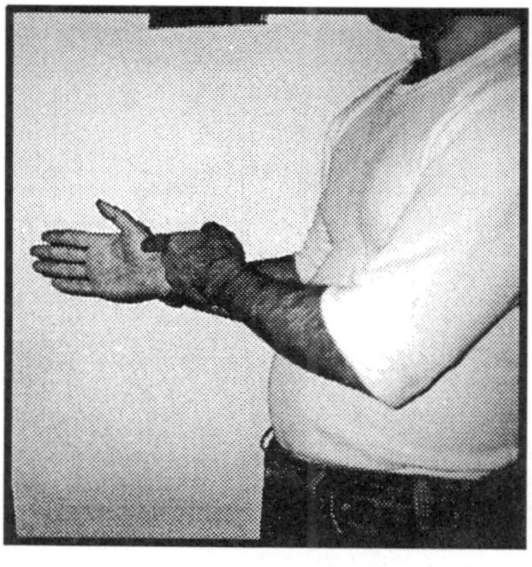

One of the most noticeable intense arthritis-type pains would be right here in the bottom meaty part of the thumb on the hand. A dull achine — irritable intense pain. I'd have to shake, twist, push and rub this muscle to ease the pain.

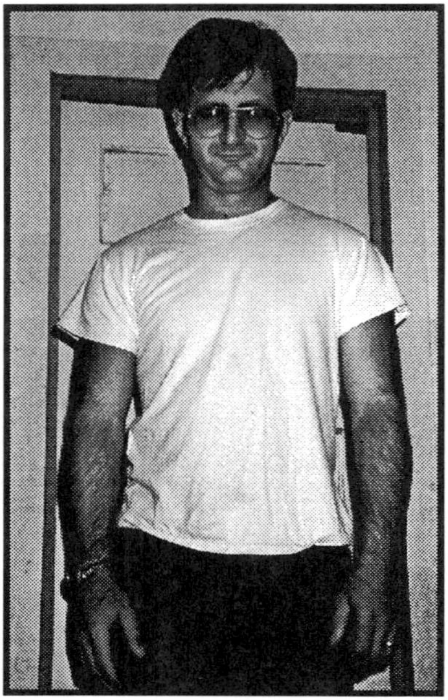

Lyme Disease
seen in the shoulder and arms

Left: Natural look without tension

Tension in the shoulder and elbow when letting one arm to do something as easily as drinking from a glass the other shoulder will lift up with tenseness and be much farther from body to counter-balance the uncoordinated feeling of the body.

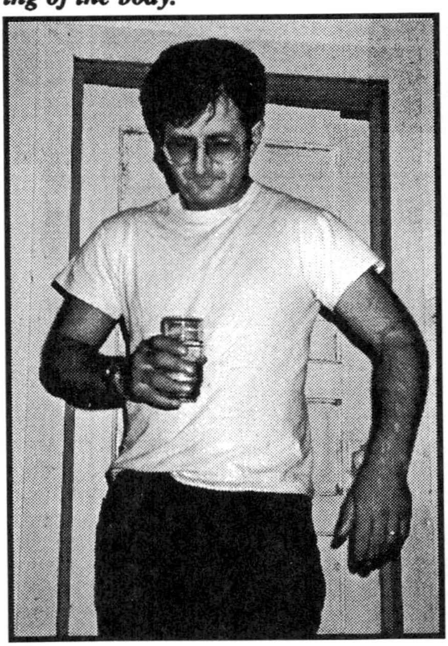

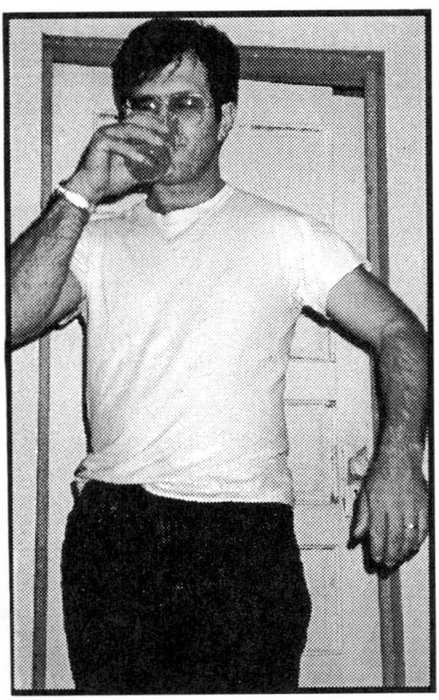

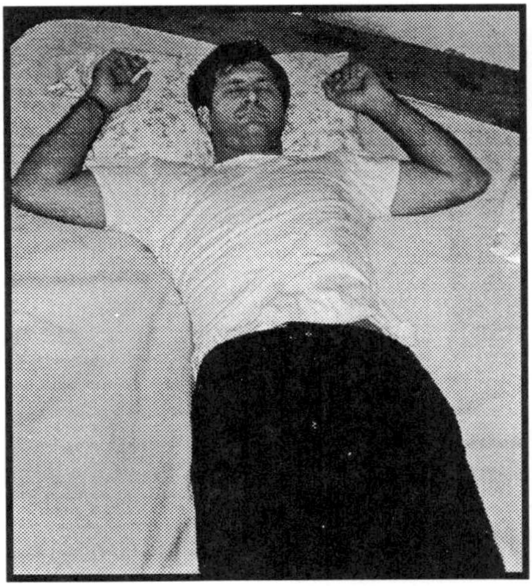
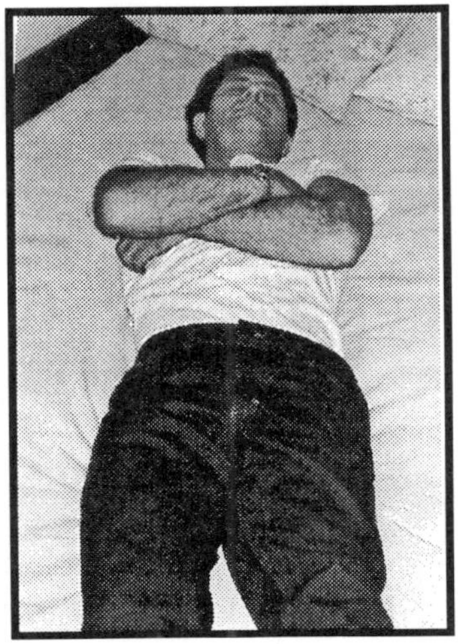
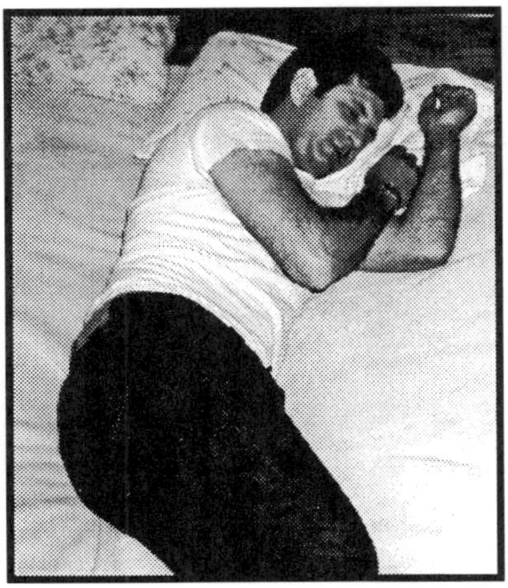
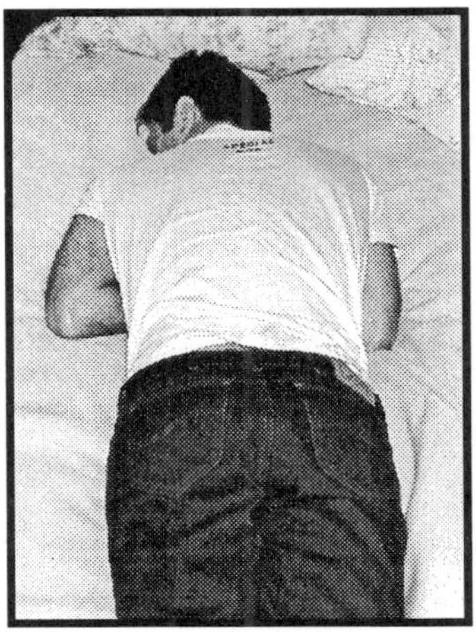

At night while sleeping, your forearms, hands and fingers will fall asleep with a numb, tingly feeling, if sleeping in any of these positions for a short period of time. After taking the medication, I could sleep for hours in any of those positions without the numb, tingly falling asleep feeling of the hands.

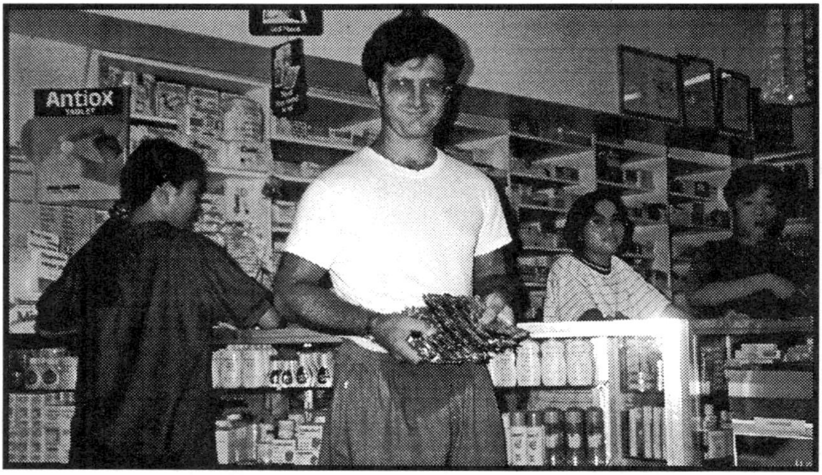

Me in a 3rd World country (Philippines) buying all the antibiotics I need to fight my disease — over the counter without a prescription.

The form of antibiotic I've found to work best and quickest is the tetracycline form, 500 mg. three times a day. Within a week you will be able to tell if you have this disease or not.

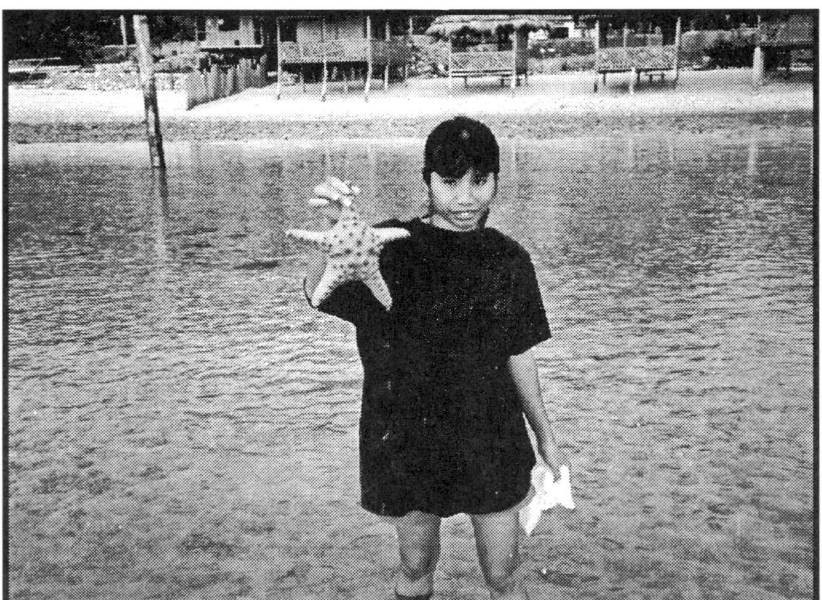

This is the little woman I found on the other side of the earth and made my wife.

LYME DISEASE SYMPTOMS IN TODDLERS

July 28, 1996, the baby is born. Eight days later he was bitten by a seed tick. When I saw that seed tick, my heart dropped. I got a sad feeling and said to myself that he is infected and at such a young age. I cried inside, understanding how the word normal was going to be missing from the baby's childhood, and not only a baby, but *my* baby's childhood. I looked at my wife, knowing she wouldn't understand either because she hadn't been bitten. (I'll try to make this story short.)

My wife said, "Come look at this mole, it grew fast."

I looked at it and said, "It's a tick."

She said, "No."

I poked at it and the legs moved. That is when my heart dropped and I said, "It's a tick." I got it off, kept it, and wiped the spot with alcohol, went to the doctor for the baby's second-week check-up, told the nurse that he was bitten by a tick and showed her the tick.

She said, "Don't worry about it. The baby has immunities to stuff at such a young age." And she also said, "Lyme disease is not around here, is it?"

I said, "Yeah, I had it."

She said, "Don't worry," but of course I did, because I know all about it. I prayed that somehow he would not be infected, but I knew in my mind that it doesn't matter how many or what kind of tick bites you, all ticks carry a form of this disease.

Months later, I could see all the symptoms in my baby, mostly in hands and fingers and rolling, avoiding eyes. I told the doctor that he had it.

The doctor said he hadn't seen many cases around here and he probably didn't have it.

I said, "Can you give him some antibiotics?"

He said, "Let's wait, he's still young."

I told my wife and friends that he had it.

They said, "Shut up, don't say that, he is okay."

I said, "No, I can tell."

I couldn't get support from anybody; everyone said to forget about it. I couldn't ignore it because we now have insurance and a doctor. With that the fight should not be so hard. What was missing was cooperation, education and a nurse or doctor who would listen and believe, and also access to medicine.

On the baby's six-month doctor's visit, they said he had an ear infection and finally gave him an antibiotic, 100 mg. of Amoxicillin three times a day. Two days later I noticed a big change in his behavior. He could smile, straighten his hands out better, looked around and started acting normal. I told the doctor's nurse about it at the next visit and asked for more antibiotics.

They said he didn't need any, he's too young. But I knew he did not take enough to be cured (only ten days' worth).

I told the doctor, "Let's take a test. We have insurance."

He said the tests aren't that good.

I said, "I know, but we have to do something. Then give him more antibiotics."

He said, "No, let's wait and see."

I said, "See what?"

He said, "See if any symptoms occur."

I said, "He already has them."

He said, "What? Swollen joints?"

I said, "No, it is in his fingers and wrist and the way he squirms and avoids eye contact."

He asked, "Are those symptoms? I don't know about that. Let's wait and see if he is uncomfortable or in pain or develops swollen joints."

I said, "That would be too late, wouldn't it?"

He said, "No, we have time."

I said, "Time for what?"

He said, "To see."

I said, "See what?"

He said to see if any symptoms occur. He wasn't cooperating, so I left, sent him a letter asking what he could do for my son and telling him that I know my son has it and that I know all about it. I sent him my news articles and book. He talked it over with his fellow pediatrician and told me that they decided to wait and see what happens.

He said, "Let us know if his joints get swollen or he is in pain."

I said, "He's only six months old; he cannot walk or talk yet. How can he tell me he's in pain when he doesn't know how to speak the word pain or understand it yet?"

When he was ten months old, we went to the Philippines. He caught an eye infection that turned out to be pinkeye and a cold. We took him to the doctor after returning to America. The nurse diagnosed him with having a cold and runny eyes from the cold.

I said, "No, his eyes are infected."

She said, "No, I think it's a cold," which again I knew it wasn't because I knew my kid.

Four days later his eyes were matted shut. I took him to the doctor, and the nurse said not to worry. They gave him an antibiotic to put in his eyes. Four days later it wasn't working. My wife and I and a couple of friends had caught it by then. The regular doctor wasn't in, so the other pediatrician came in and said it was a virus. So I told the doctor the baby also has Lyme disease. Can he have an antibiotic for that?

He looked at me and said, "Lyme disease? How do you know.?"

I said, "I have it, too." Anyway, I asked for a potent dose of antibiotic.

He said he didn't think it would help my baby's eyes, but that he might be able to use it. It was 200 mg. of some white liquid antibiotic for three times a day.

A couple of days later I noticed a big change in his attitude. He was much calmer, could look at me, smile much more and wrinkle his nose and forehead and lift his eyebrows. He had facial expressions now. About eight days after taking this antibiotic he began to stand by himself. At ten and a half months he couldn't yet stand by himself. He was wobbly legged and tender-footed. His ankle, shoulder, wrist and elbow joints stopped popping and became stronger at the joints. There wasn't any swelling, just popping at the joints. I told my wife that he was infected and needed more antibiotics.

She said, "Don't say that." She was not ready to accept that anything could be wrong with him. All she wanted was a baby; it didn't matter to her if he was perfect.

We were having trouble with our eyes, and we tried all kinds of creams and drops that didn't work, so we called in the Philippines and asked them what they used for pinkeye. It is a steroid eye drop called Pred-Forte. After seven visits to the doctor we finally got some. The problem cleared up in three days with the right medicine, and the pain and suffering were gone and we could see again. All it took was a cooperating doctor and the right medicine.

I kept telling my wife and friends that my baby had Lyme disease, but they said, "No, he doesn't." Without the support of my family it was hard, but I knew I was right. No one can fool me or get me to disbelieve what I know to be true that others don't understand. I always wanted to write a letter to the doctor to get him to understand about the symptoms and how the baby responds to antibiotics. (But I had a bad experience with writing a letters to the doctor). They put me into the mental institution, and it scared me because after I asked a lawyer what to do, the first thing he said was to stop writing letters.

So finally one days I said to myself, "Hey, I don't have to

stop writing. I need to write this doctor and tell him straight out who I am and that I need help and cooperation to help my child who is now 18 months old and suffering from arthritis, joints popping, stiffness, hyperactivity and scrambled brain.

I set up his 18-month appointment, wrote a letter to the doctor and took the baby to him. He came in, looked at my baby and said that was a very serious letter and asked what I wanted to do with the baby.

I said to give him some potent injections of antibiotics. I told the doctor I preferred him to give the baby 500 mg. of Rocephin and not just a one-time dose. I heard they used that antibiotic for chronic ear infection.

He agreed, and I told him I'd keep notes of the baby's progress. I was amazed at all that he had been suffering from. This was recorded during a 60-hour period after his first injection of 500 mg. of Rocephin.

Had injection on 1/23 at 10:30 a.m. —

5 hours after the injection of Rocephin 500 mg.

3:30 p.m., 1/23/98:

- He sits and plays without moving from the spot. Before too hyper to sit.
- Looks at you without squirming or moving. Before squirmed and moved while looking at you.
- Uses his toes to do toe stands. Before couldn't use toes very well.
- Plays with toys differently. Before didn't have time or patience to play with toys. Now he studies them using his brain.

4 p.m.:

- He is able to wrinkle his forehead and nose. Before I never saw him do that except when he took that first antibiotic 100 mg. of Amoxicillin.
- Sits and watches TV for a much longer time.
- Turns his head and can look behind himself. Before his head was stiff and always faced the front of his body.

7 p.m.

- Walk and run straight without falling down.
- Move all five toes at one time and can push with them. Before he couldn't.
- Sit and play with three things trying to figure them out. Before he couldn't sit and wasn't interested in figuring out anything. He acts like he wants to learn.
- Sits and plays with stuff a lot more. Before too hyperactive.

Next Day:

- He can walk and run in a straight line without falling. Before always walked like he was drunk.
- Looks straight into your eyes like he is thinking and knows he has a brain, too. Before, floating, nervous eyes and rapid head movement.
- Turns his head and walks or runs at the same time. Before he couldn't. The weight of his head movement would bring him down to fall.
- Sits and looks around in a real relaxed state of mind. Before, too hyper to sit and had rapid head and eye movement.
- Makes facial expressions, can move his forehead, nose, cheeks, eyebrows, ears and tongue. Before, straight-faced.
- Opens mouth much wider and leaves it open. Before he just kept his mouth shut, except to cry or eat.
- Can walk fast or run fast and stop without falling down.
- Walks on his feet more solidly. Before he wobbled like a duck.
- No more slinging his head around to move, following the weight of the movement. Before he would use the weight of his head to move in that direction. Now he uses his feet and walks there.
- Ankle joints aren't sore any more. Can stand with feet on ground and turn his head without falling. Hips and head don't sway any more when walking.
- You can lay with him by your side without all the squirming movement. Before you couldn't lay and hold him because he squirmed away. He would only lay for three seconds, then

move away. Now he just lays there and sleeps or looks around.

- No more wobble-headed movements. His head now sits straight on his shoulders.
- You can hold eye contact with him now. Before he wouldn't look at you. He was too squirmy.
- He can use all his fingers now, can lay his hand flat on a table top. He can use all fingers to hold his palm of hand off the table top. Hands aren't cold, paralyzed-looking or cramped-looking any more.
- He can separate his fingers now. Before they all stuck together and curled under.
- Now he can slap with the palm of his hand instead of slapping table tops with his wrist. Before he would use his wrist to push, hit, slap or touch with.
- No more running wildly and then falling down. Now he sits and walks.
- Eyes are much more focused, instead of rapid eye movement.

48 Hours Later

- His joints have stopped cracking and popping. Mainly wrist, ankles, shoulders don't pop any more or sound like falling apart.
- Can stand up and turn his head to the side. Before he couldn't stand and turn or walk and turn his body or head at the same time.
- Slap the table with the palm of his hand and make a slapping sound. Before he couldn't do it. He used his wrist instead of palm of hand.
- He will sit on your lap or let you hold him without fighting to be let go.
- He is a lot less squirmy before going to bed. Doesn't wake up screaming any more. Doesn't fight to lay down. Before he had too much scrambled energy to lay down.
- He eats more food. Don't have to chase him to feed him. He sits and eats and can eat by himself.
- He can walk backward without falling down. Before he

couldn't walk forward without falling down.

- Can hang his feet over a chair when sitting and swing his feet.
- His eyes have changed from looking like an American to looking like a Filipino with slanted eyes.
- Now when he falls he doesn't fall uncontrollably down. He slowly sits down.

This was the effect the antibiotic had on him in the first 60 hours after taking it. He is still improving hour by hour. This doesn't mean he is cured. It just proves what he needs to get better and that he does respond to the medicine and he is infected.

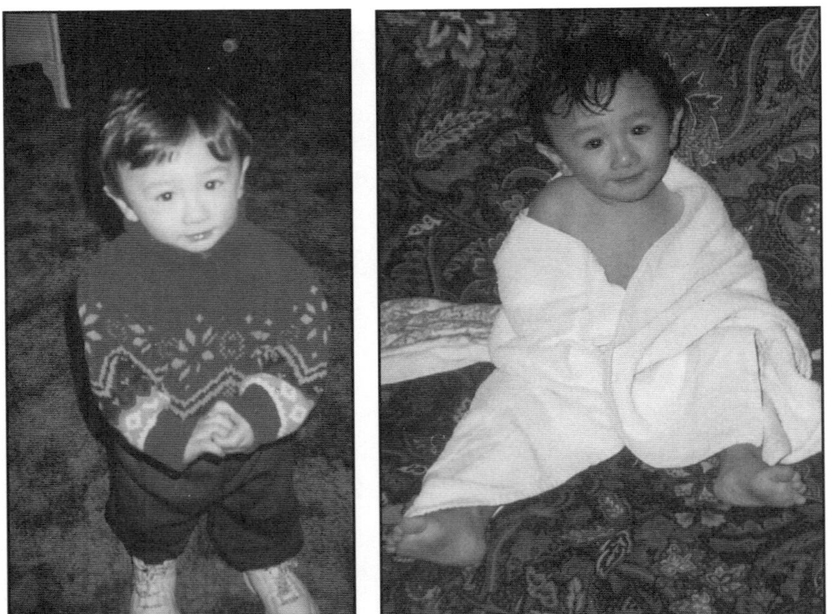

He is such a beautiful baby to have a disease that cripples his brain and body. I feel my child was sacrified so you can learn.